Learn to
Self Heal

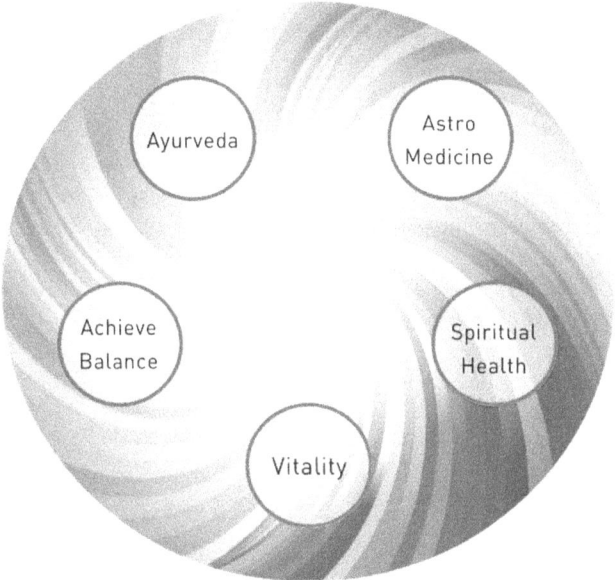

A personal and practical
approach towards wholeness

Christina Richter R.N.

Disclaimer

The information in this book is for educational purposes only. The contents herein are NOT medical advice, diagnosis or prescription. In seeking healing solutions, it is strongly advised that you work with qualified practitioners in the respective field.

Please note: It is recommended to seek professional advice from the appropriate practitioner if you wish to use herbs as part of your lifestyle as some herbs interact with prescribed medications.

The author is not responsible for damage and other liabilities.

Copyright © 2018
All rights reserved. This book or any portion thereof may not be reproduced or used in any manner whatsoever without the express written permission of the author except for the use of brief quotations in a book review.
Printed in Australia
First Printing, 2018
ISBN: 978-0-6482128-9-8
White Light Publishing
Melton, VIC, Australia 3337

whitelightpublishing.com.au

To the memory of my beloved spiritual sister Jennabeth Moss, who told me to never give up on my light. Her essence is always with me.

To Bob and Helen, who left their imprint on me and awakened my soul to mind-body health.

To Kira Sutherland, my mentor, colleague and friend who inspired me to delve into the depths of holistic health.

Contents

SECTION ONE
Astro Medicine   17
Aries   23
Taurus   28
Gemini   33
Cancer   38
Leo   43
Virgo   47
Libra   51
Scorpio   56
Sagittarius   61
Capricorn   65
Aquarius   70
Pisces   75

SECTION TWO
Simply Ayurveda   83
Vata   86
Pitta   87
Kapha   88
Dosha Test   91
Ama and Treatment   94
Four Pillars of Health   96
Nutrition   96
Tips for better digestion   97
Recipes   101
Rest   111
Relationships   112
Exercise   114
Daily Routine   116
Seasonal Support   118
How to boost energy   122

SECTION THREE
Spiritual Health   129
Chakra one   134
Chakra two   136
Chakra three   137
Chakra four   138
Chakra five   139
Chakra six   140
Chakra seven   141
Colour Meditation   142

SECTION FOUR
Modalities of Healing   147
Anne's Story   148
Aromatherapy   153
Astrobach   156
Bowen Therapy   157
Depression   159
Gestalt Therapy   165
Homeopathy   170
Māori Healing   171
Massage   173
Meditation   177
Mindfulness   181
Naturopathic Medicine   182
Pranayama   184
Rebirthing   188
Reflexology   192
Sleep   194
Tai Chi   199
Tissue Salts   202
Watsu   204
Yoga   206

Glossary   209
Acknowledgements   211

Foreword

Christina Richter has written an easy to read but comprehensive book, which is filled with valuable information and practical insights. Learn to Self-Heal will not only appeal to budding students who wish to convey their knowledge through conventional and alternative means, but it will also be alluring to those who wish to further enhance their overall knowledge of medical astrology. It is a well-written book, and it is wonderfully presented — complete with useful tips and empirical suggestions.

I particularly enjoyed the section called Modalities of Healing — containing real life case studies, which highlight the dangers of illness and disease, such as depression. The book touches briefly on the use of conventional medicines, but perhaps more importantly, and for me most impressively, it proposes the use of natural therapies as benevolent attributes towards potential healing. Currently, depression is regarded as one of the most proliferating diseases of today's modern and technological world. Furthermore, the section culminates beautifully with a collective offering of innate and spiritual attributes — denoting the importance of mindfulness, naturopathic medicine, and meditation.

I also enjoyed Christina's recipe ideas — some of which I have adopted. Overall, this is a very knowledgeable book, and within its pages, there is no doubt something that will appeal to everyone. Learn to Self-Heal is an exceptionally well written book, and it is even in its approach to the practice of medical astrology and all of the disciplines that are connected to and enhanced by it. Therefore, it is a book that I would highly recommend to others. Finally, I feel that this is a book that has been written directly from the heart.

Alan Richards-Wheatcroft
Medical Astrologer and Spiritual Healer.

Introduction
"The body speaks what the soul seeks." – Christina Richter

Welcome to my book, 'Learn to Self-heal', a personal and practical guide towards wholeness. I hope you find this information helpful and easy to implement into your daily life. My intention here is simple. I purely want to share what I have found to be supportive to my body-mind and useful over my many years in mainstream medicine, as a Registered Nurse and as a Medical Astrologer. My goal is to be of service by sharing what I have understood and learnt with my spiritual journey regarding health and may this book guide you in understanding yourself and maintaining holistic wellness.

As I reflect on this process, I realise that every time I became sick or was unwell, I was storing information and experiences that would be the foundation for me choosing a life of service.

When I was a child I suffered with red, hot pustules on my body. Yes, boils. I used to get these on my legs, my arms and my back. As a child I never spoke up or answered back to my parents and as a result I held my angry emotions inside. I understood later, as a healer, that angry emotions that have no outlet will represent themselves as eruptions on your skin. In Louise Hay's book, *You can heal your life,* boils are a symptom of anger boiling over or poisonous anger and personal injustice.

> ...angry emotions that have no outlet will represent themselves as eruptions on your skin...

As a child, I felt powerless; this was reflected in my choice of partners over the years. The relationships I had reinforced my belief that I had no personal power and, therefore, nothing important to say. The beauty of dysfunctional relationships is that these associations are often quite painful, and this pain pushes you to take action around your own life, usually for the positive. In my case, they were a catalyst for me to find my own personal power and realise that I too, have a voice that should be heard. This quest took over most of my adult life as I was learning and growing into myself.

Part of my mission in acquiring my own personal power was making decisions around my health. In my first year of nursing, I was twenty-three years old and I nursed two patients at the same time who had a profound effect on how I was starting to understand health.

> Part of my mission in acquiring my own personal power was making decisions around my health.

The first was a sixty-year-old man, who I will name Bob. Bob came into hospital for minor surgery for his ingrown toenail. We got chatting and Bob told me about his experience with abdominal cancer thirty years prior. This tweaked my interest as I believed at that time that if you were diagnosed with cancer, your life was limited.

Bob shared with me that his doctor told him that was actually the case. This was a wakeup call for him, so he took drastic steps to change his life immediately. He left his job as CEO of a major company, started a diet of whole organic foods, spent time with his family and laughed a lot more.

I was amazed. At that point, I really looked at the patient lying in the hospital bed and I asked Bob what he thought was the main thing that had saved him. Bob replied it had all helped, but for him, the love and support of his family is what encouraged him to let go of his old life which was apparently killing him, and he didn't even know it. Bob looked so light lying in the hospital bed and I could see he was a man very much at peace with life and with himself.

At the same time, I nursed a forty-seven-year-old woman whom I will call Helen, who had just been diagnosed (while in hospital) with lung cancer. The doctor informed her that she had about eighteen months of life expectancy. The news was a shock to Helen and naturally she did not take the news well. I sat with Helen during the shift and asked if she had people to support her through this time until she decided what she was going to do. Helen shared with me that she had no family, just one friend; her energy felt dark and heavy. On reflection, I feel Helen was in a deep depression that no one picked up on as the medical focus was on the cancer and not on how it was affecting her emotionally.

While I was sitting on the chair trying to console her (the best I could in my limited experience), Helen asked me to pass her scarf and some jewellery. Helen started to give them to me for being so kind to her. I refused and stated that it was against hospital policy to accept gifts and that she would be needing her items on discharge. Helen told me that she would be dead by morning and that she had no one to give her things to. I felt a pang of deep sadness at this woman's loss within herself and I replied in a cheery voice that I would see her the following day, hoping my positive attitude would lift her spirits. I left shift at 11pm and returned to work at 7am the following morning. Helen died at 6.30am that morning in her sleep.

In my nursing career when dealing with grief and loss, I would often think about Bob and Helen. I came to understand that Bob was right. He had the loving support of his wife and family which gave him a purpose and a reason to make the changes he needed to make, to live a happier and fruitful life. Helen felt alone, and although she had eighteen months of life expectancy, she felt she had no one to share her loss or her life with. So, the love and the human connectedness you have with people gives purpose to life. Helen had no purpose, therefore no reason to want to live. They both left their imprint on me in separate ways, which awakened my soul.

I am grateful to Helen and Bob as they woke me up to the power the mind has over the body, and to come to realise the choices you make can make a difference to your longevity.

At age twenty-five years, I was told I needed surgery because I had a bowel obstruction. I felt sick and was in constant, excruciating pain. Sure enough, the barium X-ray showed a twisted bowel. "Well", I thought, "that explains the agonising pain I was experiencing." I refused the surgery and told my doctor in desperation that there *must* be another way. The thought of being cut open so young and having a colostomy bag was not an option for me, not at the tender, vibrant age of twenty-five. My concern was: I will never have sex again! Who would want me with a colostomy bag? This thought was devastating.

My doctor thought about it and put me on a high fibre diet, copious fluids and strong laxatives. It took time and discipline, but it did the trick. Unknown to me at the time, that experience had planted a seed, that when it came to health and my body, I had options. I realised that I only had to ask the right question or seek them out. I did have a choice. The other realisation was that surgery is not always the only option. I have applied this

> ...when it came to health and my body, I had options... I only had to ask the right question or seek them out.

concept to various other conditions I have had over the years. It has taken longer for healing to occur, but I have avoided major surgery. Therefore, I always ask informed questions and encourage my clients to do the same when they see their doctor.

While working in intensive care, I applied to update my skills and do a wound management workshop. What attracted me to this workshop was the session on using aromatherapy in wound healing. It was the last session of a two-day workshop and it was well worth the wait. The presenter was a registered nurse with a background in aromatherapy and healing touch. She talked about how aromatherapy was beneficial for burns and how certain oils fight infection. She also referred to energy healing and how this could accelerate physical wound healing. This fascinated me. I approached her after class and she invited me to a Healing Touch seminar that was being held that weekend. Of course, as divine timing would have it, I was not working, so I attended.

Four years later, I was a qualified Healing Touch Practitioner and this knowledge gave me more insight into my own health and the disease process.

Meanwhile, I studied Colour Therapy, Stress Management, Ayurveda and Astrology. Medical Astrology seemed like a natural progression. I had a keen interest in health and the thought of identifying your body's physical weakness connected to psychological beliefs in your birth chart just seemed logical. Understanding your personal blueprint gives the knowledge you need to strengthen your health and therefore, prevent or minimise dis-ease. Once I started working on this level, illness made sense. People who had moon issues in their charts often had connection problems with their mothers. They lacked the ability to nurture themselves in a healthy manner, although they often nurtured others well. As a result, they would often suffer with digestion problems which is the seat of nurturing and most disease issues. Digestion assimilates all your nourishment from food and reflects how you digest life.

We know life's a journey and I was in the thick of it when I stumbled into Ayurveda. I was on one of my many trips to India, when my friend Vicky asked me to be her support person in her quest to be drug-free. I had never experienced anything like it. In one week, I saw a dark person literally turn almost white as the toxins were flushed out of her body. There were no chemicals involved, just the Ayurvedic process. Well I was hooked. I ventured into a six-year learning spree, like a dog with a bone, travelling between Australia and India to learn this ancient healing system.

When I was forty years old, I was diagnosed with spinal compression of my vertebra in my lower back. I was told I would not be able to pick up anything more than five kilos and that I would never be able to run again. At that time, I was due to take another trip to India to study, so I deferred any further treatment. While in class, I started to experience concentrated sharp pain in my lower back, so bad I had to stop class and lie down. In Ayurveda, pain is referred to as a Vata imbalance is a strong indicator that something was out of alignment in my body-mind. With this awareness, I decided to get my lower back healed using Ayurvedic treatments. I underwent intense therapy which included a special diet, yoga, pranayama, warm oil massage and working on my own inner demons which I needed to understand and

> *Holistic Health believes a healthy body and soul come from an unencumbered mind and body, taking ... every part of the whole body to bring the internal environment into balance...*

release. That was fifteen years ago and to this day, I have had no further problems with my back, and yes, I can lift more than five kilos and do short runs completely pain free. There is truth in the saying that what you seek, you shall find and 'where you focus your energy, you will manifest'.

The World Health Organisation states: 'Health is a state of complete physical, mental and social well-being and not merely the absence of disease or infirmity.'

Holistic Health believes a healthy body and soul come from an unencumbered mind and body, taking into consideration every part of the whole body to bring the internal environment into balance.

When you go to the doctor, they ask, "What is wrong with you?" and treat you via your symptoms. When you go to a Holistic Practitioner, they ask you what is not working in your life as a reflection of what is not working in your body. This connects the body-mind to the soul when it comes to treatment.

As a registered nurse, I have spent thirty-three years in traditional medicine specialising in intensive care. In that time, I have found conventional medicine certainly does have a significant role to play, especially in the areas of trauma and necessary surgery. A major frustration I have experienced in the medical model is that doctors and nurses often deal with people who refuse to take responsibility for their own health. They come to hospital looking for quick cures and often present the same symptoms back to their own doctor once they have returned to their unhealthy lifestyle. Having choice around body maintenance and health preservation is the aim of this book.

When your health fails, this inhibits your ability to continue being productive in the workforce, limiting income and promotion.

> *...when you are young you abuse your health to create your wealth; when older, you use your wealth to maintain your health...*

Extra emotional and monetary responsibility and stress are placed on your family and all relationships. Your future is on hold and you are stuck until you reach wellness or recovery.

What if you could identify your body's weaknesses and strengthen them? What if you were armed with the information and tools to minimise and prevent illness? What if you knew what you needed to be healthy, to live longer and be vitally strong?

Nobody is born perfect. We inherit our parents' disease patterns. This is reflected in our horoscope. It's only a matter of time before signs start to emerge to confirm this. Other influences like diet, lifestyle, pollutants, stress, psychological, emotional and environmental conditioning contribute to this loss of perfection.

In some cultures, it is customary to seek the local astrologer to define and determine a child's life purpose and predisposition to illness. The child is then raised and nurtured in accordance with their life purpose as it is outlined in the birth chart. Freewill is very much a part of this process, as every experience contributes to the outcome. As a soul, some have chosen disease as a path to dissolve karma and learn lessons more quickly during their recovery and healing, they often give back to their community as part of the process.

My definition of health is related to the element Air – from the first breath we take when we are born, to the last breath before we pass over. We cannot live without air for more than three minutes before we start to decay: our mind, body and soul. All living things have this vital Prana (air) as a form of vital energy. Without it we cannot exist.

The element of Air captures the essence of what this book is about. It represents creativity, intelligence, adaptability, information, flow of things and innate wisdom. The acronym **A.I.R.** defines this.

A   AWARENESS

Astrology and Ayurveda are used to cultivate awareness in two areas. First, the spiritual and psychological in identifying life patterns, enabling people to learn their life lessons. Secondly, the medical, in bringing forth the psychosomatic causes underlying disease and imbalance in the body.

I   INFORMATION

This book provides the education and information tailored to the individual. 'Be aware and be informed' is the mantra derived from the belief that people need to be educated in alternatives available to them, so they can choose the best options suitable for their individual needs.

R   RESPONSIBILITY

The tools offered throughout this book aim to bring balance to your life, so you are better equipped to face life's challenges.

As an evolved soul, it is your responsibility to become conscious by making correct choices that serve you and bring about your own ability to self-heal. The practitioner is only as useful as the client's willingness to take self-responsibility and make change for their own benefit.

In my capacity as a consultant, what constantly amazes me is the answers I get when I ask my clients the question, "What is most important to you in life?" In 95% of cases responses are: family, love or relationships, career, money, the future, then their health, and usually in that order. Those who have experienced a medical crisis like cancer, usually put health as the first or second most important pillar in their life. They have learned to appreciate and understand the value of their wellbeing; its paramount function as the foundation to all things around them and with what they want to achieve.

I believe we are spiritual beings choosing to have a physical experience, therefore we need to honour both our spiritual and physical needs equally. Excess or deficiency in either will bring dis-ease to the body. The part of the body affected reflects where we need to adjust our life. Pain is a symptom of something in our life not aligned to our true self. Like in Bob's story, his job was killing him, and he didn't even realise it.

As a human species, we are very fortunate that we possess a multi defence system which is called our immunity. Our first level where we fight invaders is in our mind. Our positive thoughts influence our every being, right down to cell level. What we think we are, we become. Energy goes where your focus goes... so watch what you think and how often you think that same thought or belief, e.g. being 'pissed off' usually correlates to problems with kidneys.

> ...our digestion contributes 70 percent of our immunity and works in conjunction with our liver, therefore it is important that our digestion is kept healthy...

Our second level of immunity is the auric or energy field. When our energy field is aligned with the chakras, we are grounded and in balance with our inner and outer selves. This gives us resilience, which prevents foreign bugs entering our body.

Our third line of defence is our skin. Our skin cells are replaced every 21 days and the skin is regenerated every 35 days, and this is the protective layer which keeps invaders away. So, whenever there is a break in the skin's integrity, you need to clean and cover the wound quickly to prevent unwanted and possibly harmful germs.

We also have our digestive acid and digestive enzymes, which are friendly bacteria that aid the immunity process. Our digestion contributes 70% of our immunity and works in conjunction with our liver; therefore, it is important that our digestion is kept healthy. The cells of the stomach lining and large bowel (colon), which is part of the digestion process, are renewed every four days.

www.nourishholisticnutrition.com

Part of our spleen's role is to produce and remove blood cells, which helps in supporting the immune system. Likewise, the appendix has a vital function in directing lymphocytes to aid in fighting inflammation and infection. Last but not least, we have our army of white blood cells or leucocytes whose primary role is to fight invading organisms that are harmful to the body.

We are truly magnificent in our being-ness. Not only do we hold the innate ability to prevent inflammation and infection, we can also regenerate our cells on an ongoing basis. We renew our red blood cells and liver cells every four to five months and the body can fully regenerate after five to seven years. How the body regenerates will depend on how you have lived your life in that time. So, if you have lived a life of distress, wrong action and misalignment with your passion or purpose, then your body is programmed accordingly. Likewise, the reverse.

In conclusion, this is not new information. There are hundreds of therapists and healers out there using ancient wisdoms and modern treatments to treat dysfunction in the body-mind. All I have done is share my journey and hope it will enable you to use this information to maintain your health, and to have choice around your wellbeing journey towards wholeness.

Christina Richter © 2018

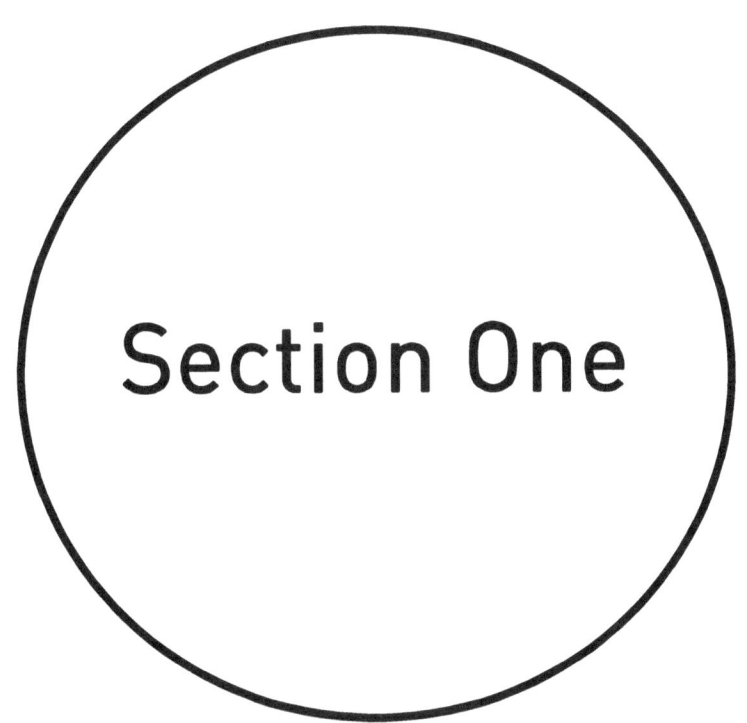

Section One

Astro-Medicine

"A physician without the knowledge of astrology cannot rightly call himself a physician." Hippocrates (460-357BC) the Father of Modern Medicine.

What is Astro-medicine?

Astro-medicine is the marriage of the ancient healing art of astrology and the mysteries of medicine. The focus here is on self-understanding, prevention and body maintenance, resulting in self-healing. Complementary medicine holds a greater priority here as these therapies are usually holistic and integrated in its methodology. Modern medicine does have a role to play in healing and should not be disregarded if the need arises; if anything, it can work effectively in conjunction with other therapies. Seek medical advice if you are on life sustaining medication.

...your Astrology chart is your blueprint of life...

How to determine your imbalance in your personal horoscope?

Your Astrology chart is your blueprint of life. This powerful insightful tool reveals all. With significant accuracy, your personal birth chart will identify your personality, psychological lessons, spiritual direction, karma, career focus, financial capacity, and love analysis, in which city to buy a house, your fertility and naturally, your health. Who would have thought that all this is determined the moment you take your first breath? Pretty amazing don't you think?

Astro-medicine is the integrated science which will identify your body constitution, metabolism and ailments relating to psychological, spiritual, emotional and mental disharmony.
Your healing potential in combination with a personal plan for living in harmony with yourself and your environment is also highlighted. As a result, this information if put into daily practice, will strengthen your constitution while maintaining health and therefore minimising or preventing further disease.

Now, why should you believe all this?

Early astronomers also used astrology. In fact, astrology was known as the mother of astronomy.

In his book *Astrology, the Evidence of Science,* Dr Percy Seymour, a renowned astronomer and astrophysicist, reveals how the central nervous system is affected by magnetic fields. Science has now shown the universe to be a complex system of electromagnetic forces.

As you may know, our living auras are electromagnetic fields which exist in our auric/spiritual body. This is connected through a subtle energy system of chakras that are connected by channels called *nadis*. This chakra system directly affects our physical body via the endocrine system and central nervous system.

Psychologist and statistician Michael Gauquelin, over forty years, assembled a study of 25,000 individuals spread across nine professions, from five countries. He found a striking correlation between planetary influences at birth and the choice of occupation. There was a strong relationship between moon placement and certain personality traits. He lists these in his book, *The Truth about Astrology*.

How to read your own horoscope

What I am about to show you here is a very simple formula for you to identify areas of health that need strengthening. Be mindful that a more comprehensive analysis is far more complex, and a session is usually 1 ½ - 2 hours long.

The word horoscope is from the Greek word *horoskopos* with *hora* meaning 'hour' and *skopos* meaning 'watching'.

In Medical Astrology, three planets: The Sun, Moon, Saturn and the ascendant, will identify most medical ailments for a person. The ascendant is formed at the time of birth of the person. If you do not have a time of birth, this does not prevent you from having a workable chart. You can obtain a birth time from your family, birth certificate, hospital records, or through muscle testing.

First, you need a birth chart. For this you need your date, time and city of birth. If you do not have a chart, go to www.astro.com or email me on crscorpio1111@gmail.com with these details and a free chart will be given to you. Your date of birth correlates to your Sun Sign and you can use the information in this book to strengthen your body constitution and increase your vitality. This is an excellent place to start. Print out your chart and put it aside for the moment.

Secondly, you need to understand the astrological signs, as this is how they will appear on your chart. They are as follows:

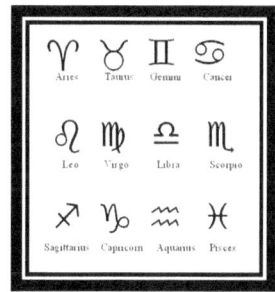

Next you need to identify the following in your chart.

Ascendant: This is determined by the *time* you were born. Your ascendant describes your typical characteristics and disposition. It also rules your first house in your chart that defines your physical body and any potential illness relating to it.

Sun: This is represented by your *date* of birth, e.g. 11th November makes you a Scorpio. Your Sun sign determines your physical vitality and health. Also, the Sun reveals how you shine in the world and signifies father and male authority figures in your life.

Moon: This represents your soul memory, emotional nature and your bodily fluids. The Moon also signifies mother or mother figures in your life.

Saturn: Is the karmic lord of the chart and is also known as Father Time. He represents the lesson you need to learn to evolve to your full potential. Also, this is where obstacles or blockages need to be identified and strengthened in relation to life and to health.

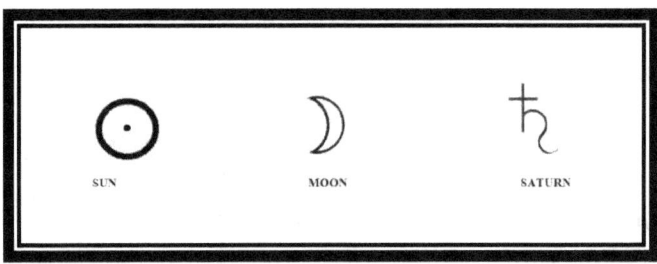

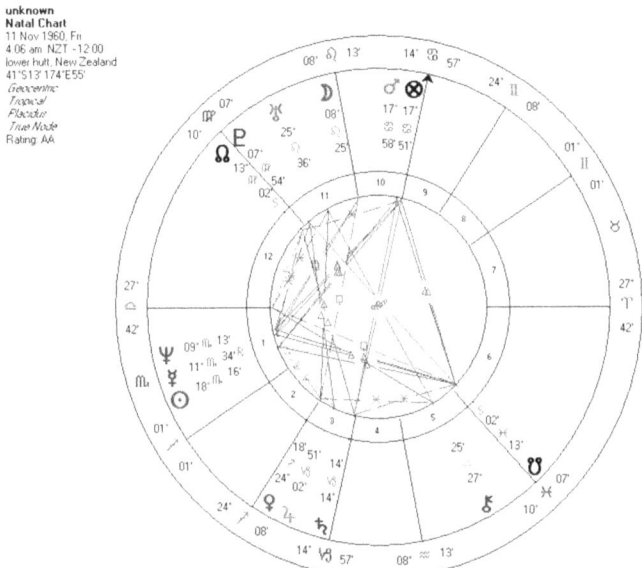

Practical example

This is a typical astrology chart in the western system.

<u>First identify the Ascendant</u>: LIBRA 27 degree 42' and read the section relating to Libra

<u>Second identify the Sun:</u> SCORPIO 18 degree 16' and read the section relating to Scorpio

<u>Next identify the Moon</u>: LEO 8 degree 25' and read the section relating to Leo

<u>Last identify Saturn</u>: CAPRICORN 14 degree 14' and read the section relating to Capricorn the *affected body section, disease and ailments and treatments sections only.*

Now read the sections on Leo, Libra, Scorpio and Capricorn (as relevant to the chart above).

21

Please remember that because this is only a small part of the overall interpretation (about 25%) that this is a guide only. As you read each section not all the information will apply to you, although some of it will be spot on. You will recognize parts of yourself in what you read, and it will just feel right. We all have intuition which comes from our soul, and this cannot lie, always trust it. Take what applies to you only.

Naturally the other planets and houses are involved in Astro-diagnosis, but for the purpose of this book and for non-astrologers we will keep it simple and just use Sun, Moon, Saturn and the ascendant.

Now apply this formula to your own chart and use the personal notes at the end of this chapter to write your findings.

Remember, if you do cannot obtain a birth time, use your date of birth and read the sign associated with it e.g. if born on 1st January then you are a Capricorn. The sun-sign is the most vital part of the chart when it comes to vitality and health.

ARIES   Me, myself and I

Ruler: Mars   **Element:** Fire   **Mode:** Cardinal

Personality Profile

Arians are action oriented and are known as the Warrior in the zodiac, eager to experience new things and often initiating new projects. When energies are scattered, projects are not usually seen through to completion. Aries are spontaneous by nature and will often make risky decisions without thinking things through. Pioneers and visionaries in their field, they are brilliant and make natural leaders.

When balanced, Arians are positive, dynamic, courageous, independent, daring, optimistic and adventurous in their endeavours.

When unbalanced they become impatient, inconsiderate of others, thoughtless, self-centred, stubborn and do not take responsibility for their actions or in some cases non-action.

Aries will often create and carry a self-defeatist attitude. They may choose to lack self-control and understanding of any given situation, projecting all blame onto others. Once they take control and develop understanding of their own path in life, they will then shine like the beacon of light they are destined to be.

> *Once they take control and develop understanding of their own path in life, they will shine like a beacon of light...*

Affected Body Systems
- Muscular system
- Body parts affected include brain, skull, head, face, eyes, ears, sinus, adrenal gland, pituitary gland and blood.

Disease and Ailments
Ruled by Mars the planet of raw energy and physical drive, you can push yourself to exhaustion. Daily physical outlet is required as you usually have an excess of energy. If you are involved in competitive sports, you may deplete your adrenal system and overtax your nervous system which will affect your brain. If Aries is lacking a physical outlet they will then become emotional and will express themselves with the following mannerisms: frustration leading to irritability, being quick tempered, aggressive and sometimes angry. Other symptoms may be exhibited as feelings of impulsiveness and being accident prone.

Harbouring thoughts of depression accompanied by self-doubt, feelings of guilt, being self-centred, ungrounded, with unsound risky decision making are not uncommon. It is best for Aries to express their energy in the morning; this is when they are most active. Aries often have high fevers and tend to recover from illness quickly.

Aries primarily rules the head; Arians are prone to conditions affecting this area. Congestion and inflammation are common. Ailments include headaches, earaches, epilepsy, neuralgia, dizziness, nosebleeds, ailments to eyes, ears and nose, insomnia, high blood pressure, hair loss, hay-fever and scars.

Nutrition Nourishing

Helpful foods include whole grains, dark green leafy vegetables, brewer's yeast, nuts, mushrooms, fish, dates, parsley, dried apricots, and blackstrap molasses. As Aries are fiery, cooling foods like strawberries, dates, apples, grapefruit, tomatoes, celery, cabbage, beetroot, cucumbers, watercress, spinach, lettuce and asparagus can be very soothing. Foods high in iron such as meats, turkey and fish are best as Aries need extra iron due to high activity.

Spicy, heating foods should be avoided, as should stimulants e.g. caffeine, tea, chocolate, alcohol as this will over stimulation of the nervous system.

Foods containing essential vitamins suitable for Aries:

A: Liver, carrots, parsley, sweet potato, spinach, mangos, chives, tomatoes and broccoli.

B12: Liver, beef, chicken, oysters, scallops, fish and cottage cheese.

C: Citrus fruits, red chilli peppers, kale, parsley, cauliflower, broccoli, turnip greens, spinach, cabbage, mangos, oysters, lima beans, strawberries and raspberries.

D: Fish liver oils, tuna, salmon, sardines and dairy.

Folic Acid: Chicken and beef livers, asparagus, lettuce, broccoli, fresh orange juice, legumes and dark leafy green vegetables.

Helpful Herbs
- Burdock as a blood cleanser.
- Oats, Skullcap, Passionflower and Valerian to aid in soothing the Central Nervous System.
- Rosemary, Ginkgo and Brahmi for memory.
- Gota Kola and Ashwagandha are also beneficial for soothing nerves.
- Horseradish and garlic for sinus.

Minimising Stress
Aries do well to channel excess energy into sports, preferably in the morning: running, martial arts, competitive sports, team sports, boxing, swimming, the gym, tennis, water sports and other adventurous activities.

Avoid wearing the colour red, drinking coffee and other caffeine-based beverages, alcohol and eating spicy foods that stimulate. Wear blues and greens to promote calmness, drink plenty of water to keep cool and well hydrated, maintain a regular daily routine and eat every few hours as you burn up energy very fast. Be actively focused when achieving your goals.

Spiritual Chakra Manipura
Aries is ruled by Mars, the God of War. It is quite natural for Arian types to be concerned with issues of power related to their own sense of self. This third chakra is located at the solar plexus and relates to ego, personal power, autonomy, physical energy, metabolism, drive, courage and personal will. This gives a strong self-esteem and self-respect when in balance.

Signs of imbalance include ulcers, allergies, digestive disorders, liver and gallbladder ailments, low vitality, misplaced anger, and control issues, sensitivity to criticism, low self-esteem, introversion and shame.

Therapeutic Treatments

Bach Remedy: Impatiens

Will help Arians to develop tolerance for those who are not as dynamic as they are and will give Arians the ability to slow down and work with co-workers and family productively.

Signature Oil: Rosemary
Rosemary is warming and stimulating in nature. Particularly good for the head and brain, it is excellent in treating headaches, sinusitis and catarrh. Also used for refreshing a tired mind and improves memory.

Vibration Colour: Bright Red

When feeling positive - assertive, passionate, alert, dynamic, warm and strong.

When feeling negative – exhausted, angry, impatient, weak-willed and impractical and wearing blue and greens gives more balance.

Karmic Purpose
To understand you are here to learn about yourself. To do so successfully, you must learn to share and be considerate of others. What you see in the other is often lessons you need to learn in yourself.

Affirmation - 'Every day in every way I feel energized, assertive and alive.'

TAURUS   Solid as a Rock

Ruler: Venus   **Element:** Earth   **Mode:** Fixed

Personality Profile

Taurus is security oriented and is known as the Connoisseur in the zodiac. They are reliable, determined, solid and loyal by nature, and are admired by others because of these qualities. Taurus excels as a person when they have security in all things. They are happy to make a commitment in a relationship if this relationship has a solid foundation.

Likewise, when they have their own home, they feel safe. Renting is not a preference, not if they can own their own home. Their home is the place they go to relax. Their home will be very natural with wood interiors that reflect the sturdiness of their personality.

Gourmet food, wine, clothes, art and antiques will be part of their home décor and furniture.

When balanced, Taureans are reliable, patient, practical and admire the planet in all its abundance and beauty.

When unbalanced, Taurus becomes bull headed, not listening to anyone. Being rigid in their decision can keep them stuck in a rut. When this happens they lack motivation, become introvert and are prone to laziness.

Affected Body Systems
- Metabolic system
- Hormonal system
- Body parts affected: neck, tonsils, throat, pharynx, vocal cords, thyroid glands, shoulders, cervical vertebra,

lower jaw, base of brain, kidneys, and muscles in the shoulders.

Disease and Ailments
Ruled by Venus the planet of balance, its function is homeostasis in the body through the hormonal system and endocrine system.

Taurus primarily rules the throat and is prone to conditions affecting this area. Sore throats and stiffness in the neck and shoulders are common. Ailments include glandular fever, laryngitis, tonsils, and thyroid disease. Taurus can also suffer with constipation and haemorrhoids.

As a Taurus, you are inclined to contain your emotions and if not released constructively, this will manifest as illness. You can become stubborn when it comes to your health. You tend to delay when it comes to seeking medical advice if you suspect that you are ill. This is foolhardy as you eventually end up in the doctor's office, usually with more severe symptoms. Prevention is cure. Body maintenance will keep you away from the hospital.

> *As a Taurus you are inclined to contain your emotions and if not released constructively, this energy will manifest as illness.*

Nourishing Nutrition
Beneficial foods include: seaweed, green leafy vegetables, seafood, spinach, cabbage, cucumber, celery, radishes, onion, pumpkin, peaches, beans, potatoes, apples, blackberries, pomegranate, strawberries and chlorella; soy products also help thyroid regulation; drink at least 2-3 litres of water daily.

Iodine is needed to support the thyroid and metabolic system. Reliable sources include kelp, seaweed and iodized salt. Excess sugar, starch and dairy should be avoided.

Care needs to be taken not to indulge in food as a means of emotional security, especially rich foods that cause weight gain.

Foods containing essential vitamins suitable for Taurus:

B6:   Lean meat, poultry, fish, eggs, whole-wheat breads and cereals, nuts, bananas, soybeans, brown rice, lentils, lima beans, avocados, spinach, potatoes, cauliflower, popcorn and leeks.

E: Vegetable oil, wheat germ, soybeans, whole grains, raw nuts, raw seeds and eggs.

Niacin: Lean meat, pulses, poultry, potatoes, salmon, tuna, peanuts, liver, beef, veal, mushrooms, brown rice and dried peaches.

Helpful Herbs

- Trikatu an Ayurvedic herb that stimulates metabolism
- Gymnema blocks the intestinal absorption of sugar and regulates blood sugar levels
- Slippery elm, Kelp, and Fenugreek - support the thyroid gland

Minimising Stress
For Taurus, regular exercise is required to maintain weight. Wearing yellow and orange will stimulate activity when you feel stuck or unmotivated. Adding hot spices to diet will promote metabolism and therefore aid digestion. As you love to wind

down after work, playing peaceful music in a serene environment will satisfy the soul. You probably have a golden voice so singing to your heart's content will not only soothe your soul but will also strengthen your immunity. As you are a very tactile person, sacred stone massage therapy and head and shoulder oil massage will make you feel good and centred. Both are Ayurvedic Therapies.

Spiritual Chakra Anahata

Venus rules the heart. This fourth chakra and is about the relationship you have with yourself, your sense of personal values, self-acceptance and self-compassion. Only when this is achieved, can you extend real love to others.

Signs of imbalance: all heart related diseases, high blood pressure, mistrust, holding onto past hurts, melancholy, grief and being unable to give and receive freely.

Therapeutic Treatments

Bach Remedy: Gentian

Will dissolve your negative outlook to life and encourage you to achieve your desired outcomes.

Signature Oil: Rose

Rose is known as the 'Queen of Oils' and is an aphrodisiac, is stimulating, an antidepressant and carminative by nature. It specifically benefits your heart and chest area, improving your sense of value, love, self-worth and inner security.

Vibration colour: Pink

When feeling positive - calming, soothing, increases confidence, affectionate, harmonious and loving.

When feeling negative - smothering, sickly, overwhelmed and stagnant.

Karmic Purpose
To establish an unshakable, grounded and valued sense of inner security to obtain external security.

Affirmation - 'I am full of confidence with an abundance of love for myself and others.'

GEMINI   Two sides to every story

Ruler: Planet Mercury   **Element:** Air   **Mode:** Mutable

Personality Profile

Gemini is intellectually oriented and is known as the Communicator in the zodiac. Gemini's desire is to learn. Curious by nature, they have a need to understand and gather as much information as they can. Having full understanding of a subject gives them a sense of security. Once this information is acquired, it needs direction for it to be of value. Often this stays in the library of the mind where its value is only to the Gemini. Knowledge was made to be shared, so they should extend their mind to others.

By nature, Geminis are also very social animals. They are at ease and comfortable in most social circles. They can adapt easily with wit and humour to any situation. They are nervous, quick, changeable, moody, scattered and restless by nature. Variety really is the spice of life for them. By achieving this they will maintain harmony in life.

Hands are an extension of the brain; therefore, Geminis tend to work well with them. Learning and receiving body massage is very therapeutic for them. Not only is it a pleasurable experience, but also very grounding.

Affected Body Systems
- Central Nervous System
- Respiratory system
- Body parts affected include lungs, trachea, bronchi, diaphragm, fingers, hands, arms, shoulders, collar bone, thymus, nerves, thoracic spine and bones of the

thoracic. Oxygenation of the blood is also under this influence.

Disease and Ailments
Ruled by Mercury the planet of intellectual and internal body communications, you tend to exhaust your nerves through over stimulation of your brain. Gemini rules the respiratory system including lungs, thoracic cavity, collarbones, the trachea, arms, hands, fingers and central nervous system. Gemini people commonly suffer from: nervous disorders, epilepsy, insomnia, anxiety, migraines, bronchitis, pneumonia, shallow breathing, and asthma, fractures of collarbones, arms, hands and general aches and pains.

Having a very busy lifestyle, you do not consider your health to be of importance. It is difficult for you to maintain regular exercise or a routine that benefits you. You can forget to eat when your mind gets distracted. You tend to eat on the go and are attracted to junk food as an easy instant fix to fuel your overtaxed mind. In the long term, this lifestyle is detrimental for your health and prohibits your ability to function mentally at your best.

> *Having a very busy lifestyle, you do not consider your health to be of importance.*

Gemini needs to have adequate sleep to recuperate from their daily activities. Most Geminis sleep with the window open for air.

Nourishing Nutrition
Beneficial foods include: root vegetables, cheese, broccoli, cauliflower, corn, apricots, peaches, pineapple, nuts, seeds, eggs, sunflower seeds, sesame seeds, tomato, mushroom, carrot, butter beans, asparagus, lecithin, and essential fatty

acids, green leafy veggies, green beans, turnips, lettuce, liquid chlorophyll, chamomile tea, broccoli, almonds, prunes, wheat germ, figs, watercress, and parsley. Limit grains and dairy as they form mucus affecting the lungs.

Foods containing essential vitamins suitable for Gemini:

B1: Pork, liver, heart, kidneys, fish, potatoes, nuts, pulses, rice bran, soy milk, rolled oats, lima beans, peas, lentils and mung beans.

B12: Liver, beef, chicken, oysters, scallops, fish and cottage cheese.

C: Citrus fruits, red chilli peppers, kale, parsley, cauliflower, broccoli, turnip greens, sprouts, spinach, cabbage, mangos, oysters, lima beans, strawberries and raspberries.

D: Fish liver oils, tuna, salmon, sardines and dairy.

Helpful Herbs

- Garlic and Echinacea to improve the immune system
- Elecampane for protection of the lungs
- Skullcap to strengthen and relax the nervous system; Brahmi and Ashwagandha to soothe the nervous system
- Liquorice to support the adrenal glands (contraindicated in high blood pressure)
- Melissa to aid in the digestive process

Minimising Stress
Gemini needs plenty of fresh air to soothe their highly active nervous systems. Activities that suit their constitution on a regular basis include ice skating, tennis, badminton, dancing, gymnastics, sprinting, skiing, yoga, meditation, swimming and

Tai Chi. As they can usually manage many things at the same time it is not uncommon for them to part-take in more than one sport. As mentioned above, eating root vegetables daily will keep them grounded. Wearing greens and earth colours will calm their nerves and keep them focused. They need intellectual stimulation so should keep a daily journal; matching their wits against others in board games and card games suits them. Debates are also good for them – so, start up a debate team.

Regular oil massage and Shirodhara therapy (an Ayurvedic therapy) keeps Gemini balanced.

Spiritual Chakra Vishuddha
Mercury rules the throat chakra, the fifth chakra, and Geminis love to socialize and be known for the knowledge they gather. This chakra governs communication, speaking and honouring your truth, choice and freewill.

Signs of imbalance include speech impediments, sore throat, cough, neck problems, laryngitis, thyroid imbalance, respiratory and/or hearing problems and lies.

Therapeutic Treatments

Bach remedy: Cerato

Will accept and access your own inner knowing, will trust your own life experience to make choices that are beneficial for their own progress.

Signature Oil: Basil

Basil is mentally stimulating, antispasmodic, cephalic (clears congestion in the head), antibacterial oil which suits the Gemini constitution well. It helps bring harmony to the mind and calms the nerves.

Vibration Colour: Green

When feeling positive - harmonious, balanced, sharing, protective and secure.

When feeling negative - insincere, selfish, jealous, threatened and insecure.

Karmic Purpose
To communicate in a clear, honest and an open manner without being misunderstood.

Affirmation – 'I am objective, centred and secure in my emotions.'

CANCER   Home is where the heart is

Ruler: Moon   **Element:** Water   **Mode:** Cardinal

Personality Profile

Cancer by nature is known to be nurturing and nourishing, primarily to others. Family and children are especially important and so is the role of being a parent. You are sensitive, romantic, emotional, protective, sentimental and self-contained. You usually make your decisions based on what emotional state you are currently feeling. This will change depending on your moods, which fluctuate often. You are ruled by the Moon, so you need to be aware that every month, two or three days before the full moon, you will become super sensitive and extra emotional. No major decisions or activities should be made at this time as your decisions will be clouded. As the full moon passes you will feel normal again.

You feel secure when you have a strong and safe home. The saying, 'my home is my haven' really applies to you. If your home is disturbed in any way, so is your mental, emotional and physical disposition.

Co-dependency and attachment can be an issue for you. You need to learn to let go of beliefs, people, foods and clothes that no longer serve you. In the disguise of security, you can become a hoarder, which clutters your ability to be an integrated person. This will affect your health, especially your digestive system which reflects how you are assimilating life.

Affected Body Systems
- Lower Digestion System.
- Body parts affected include digestion system, stomach, breasts, sternum, pancreas, salvia, blood and plasma,

gallbladder, uterus, vertebral discs, pericardium, and synovial joints.

Disease and Ailments
Ruled by the Moon you are receptive and intuitive. The Moon governs your mind, soul and soft tissues of the body. As your energy is often focused towards others, you often ignore your own needs. In time, this shows in your body, usually the stomach area. You need regular exercise to maintain your weight and keep your health.

Cancer rules the stomach, breasts, uterus, pericardium, and gall bladder. Common ailments include: digestive ailments, fluid retention, stomach ulcers, mal-absorption, gall stones, gastric mucus, coughs, physical symptoms brought on by emotional imbalance, worry and nervousness, uterine disorders. When hurt, you find comfort in food. As a consequence, you are prone to emotional overeating, which will eventually lead to obesity.

> *As your energy is often focused towards others, you often ignore your own needs.*

Nourishing Nutrition
Beneficial foods include: fresh fruit & vegetables, goat's milk, cottage cheese, eggs, rye, fish, citrus fruit, papaya, peppermint, steamed or lightly cooked foods, bananas, apricots, figs, kidney beans, lentils, spinach, sweet potato, sardines, seeds, parsley, kelp and molasses.

Avoid eating cakes and pastries, eating as a source of emotional nourishment, and eating when worried or anxious as digestion may become disturbed.

Foods containing essential vitamins suitable for Cancer:

A: Liver, carrots, parsley, sweet potato, spinach, mangos, chives, tomatoes and broccoli.

B2: Milk, yoghurt, eggs, meat, poultry, fish, liver, almonds, mushrooms, millet, parsley, cashew nuts, lentils, avocados, rye, broccoli, mung beans and asparagus.

C: Citrus fruits, red chilli peppers, kale, parsley, cauliflower, broccoli, turnip greens, sprouts, spinach, cabbage, mangos, oysters, lima beans, strawberries and raspberries.

Helpful Herbs

- Chamomile calms the nerves and is a mild digestive.
- Slippery elm will soothe digestion if inflamed.
- Raspberry leaf aids in conception.
- Peppermint and spearmint to aid digestion.
- Poke root is suitable for lumpy breasts.

Minimising Stress

Cancer loves the water. You need a water environment as this will feed your creativity and intuition. Being involved in water sports like swimming, diving, sailing, surfing and water polo really satisfies your soul.

Wearing colours of yellow and orange will promote self-esteem and self-expression. You need to surround yourself with positive people that **do not** need any mothering. This will help to develop a strong sense of personal identity.

As you are strongly creative, an artistic outlet is a great tool to express your inner personality. You need to learn to channel some of the caring, nurturing energy that you give others and pamper yourself more.

Invest in yourself and have weekly facials, massages and spa treatments. Listen to soothing music while you work, this will really chill you out.

Spiritual Chakra Ajna

Known as the brow, this is the sixth chakra; its role is linking you to your sense of knowing or intuition, wisdom, emotional intelligence, psychic awareness, dreams and visions. Cancers have a natural ability of knowing, they just need to learn to trust it. It also allows you to see the big picture clearly with a positive outlook.

Signs of imbalance include headaches, problems with your central nervous system, vision problems, hallucinations and illusions.

Therapeutic Treatments

Bach remedy: Clematis.

Very grounding and brings you back into your body. Helps you to focus on daily life and engage in with your environment.

Signature Oil- Blue Chamomile

Blue Chamomile is the 'mothering oil'. It is calming, soothing, gentle, analgesic, sedative, antispasmodic and digestive. Works well with all ailments related to the stomach and is gentle enough to use on infants and children.

Vibration Colour: White

When feeling positive - cleanliness, innocence, purity, aura protection.

When feeling negative - clinical, cold, detachment, sterile and lifeless.

Karmic Purpose
To be able to understand nurturing, it can only be successful once you have learned to nurture yourself. Only then do you have the energy to nurture others.

Affirmation − 'I surround my aura and body with the spiritual white light of protection.'

LEO   The lion's roar

Ruler: Sun   **Element:** Fire   **Mode:** Fixed

Personality Profile

Leos are fiery; creative and regal. They are known as the 'Boss' in the zodiac, so you can imagine the performance when they are not in charge. They are born to be 'King' or 'Queen', but this comes when it is well earned and deserved, and not before. Leos are not unaccustomed to striving for what they want. By nature, they are determined, confident, proud, charismatic, passionate, joyful, enthusiastic, demanding and stubborn in achieving their goals.

Your sense of personal identity is directly linked to what you achieve. When you are praised, and your achievements are validated, you excel in your performance, having the ability to outshine others. When you are not praised, you feel undervalued and this can bring on depression leading to a lack of motivation in all areas of life. Learn to develop self-approval and self-validation in all you do.

You are generous and affectionate and love to do things on a grand scale. You are keen to share your outcomes and creative ideas with others. By doing this, it will empower you and bring confidence to others. Once you are fully integrated, you are a shining source of light. Give from the heart.

Affected Body Systems
- Cardiac system and circulatory system.
- Body parts affected include heart, spleen, spinal column including its nerves and marrow, pancreas, thoracic spine and blood.

Disease and Ailments

Leo is ruled by the Sun and this governs the strength and vitality of your heart. Other body parts include the spinal column, and thoracic spine. Common ailments include all heart related ailments, palpitations, aneurysms from stress, sunstroke, muscular rheumatism, chest pain, fainting, high and low blood pressure, hardening of the arteries, and thoracic back pain.

Leos have a strong body constitution. You can recuperate quickly because of your constitution and because you don't like being sick. So, your self-determination and will can drive you to wellness. As you like to live a lavish lifestyle, overindulgence in the 'wrong' foods are the main culprit.

> *As you like to live a lavish lifestyle, overindulgence in the 'wrong' foods are the main culprit*

This will weaken your heart. As you also give from the heart, any blocks to creativity and any emotional pain related to loss or a lack of joy will also contribute to heart disease. Maintaining a strong integrity will strengthen your heart; conversely, having a weak sense of self will diminish the ability of your heart to function well.

Nourishing Nutrition

Beneficial foods include: kelp, bran, carob, buckwheat, molasses, seafood, sunflower seeds, green vegetables, chlorophyll, nuts, lean red meat, plums, beetroot, carrot, oranges, oats, asparagus, spinach, eggs, mangoes and apples. Avoid stimulants, refined, processed and overheating foods.

Foods containing essential vitamins suitable for Leo:
A: Liver, carrots, parsley, sweet potato, spinach, mangos, chives, tomatoes and broccoli.
C: Citrus fruits, red chilli peppers, kale, parsley, cauliflower, broccoli, turnip greens, sprouts, spinach, cabbage, mangos, oysters, lima beans, strawberries and raspberries.

D:	Fish liver oils, dairy, tuna, salmon, and sardines.

E:	Vegetable oil, wheat germ, soybeans, whole grains, raw nuts, raw seeds and eggs.

Helpful Herbs
- Digitalis which strengthens the heart muscle.
- Valerian high in Magnesium which supports the nervous system.
- Dill, fennel, mint, parsley, saffron and chamomile as teas or added to diet.
- Motherwort is a cardiac tonic.
- Hawthorne is a strong antioxidant for the heart.

Activities to Minimise Stress
Leos do well being outdoors and exposed to plenty of sunshine. Like a typical lion, you love to just lie in the sun and be plain lazy at times. This only becomes counterproductive when it becomes a habit. You love action and regular exercise. Running, riding, wrestling, yoga, football and weight lifting are excellent ways to channel that excess energy of yours.

Being very artistic, having an outlet for creative ideas calms the drama queen (or king) in you. Suitable outlets include photography, film, acting, music, painting, jewellery design, drama and dance. You love socializing and sharing your good fortune and graces with close supportive friends and family. Having fun relaxes you and spending time with children connects you to your inner child. Be joyous.

Spiritual   Chakra Sahasrara
Positioned at the top of the head, the seventh chakra is known to connect you to your higher self, universal truth, expanded consciousness and spiritual wisdom. Ruled by the sun, this is the total integration point of yourself aligned with soul self.

Signs of imbalance include confusion, depression, obsessive behaviour, an inability to learn, issues with attachment, epilepsy and dementia.

Therapeutic Treatments

Bach remedy: Vervain

You will experience being more tolerant of others, flexible in your views and be more of a positive role model for others.

Signature Oil: Jasmine

Jasmine is known as the 'King of Oils' and is an aphrodisiac, antidepressant, moisturising and cooling for the Leos fiery temperament. Brings about balance, confidence and assists in moving through the darkness into the sunshine.

Vibration Colour: Gold

When feeling positive - happy, intelligent, logical, optimistic, forgiving, light.

When feeling negative - irrational, heavy, sad, nervous, vindictive, disorderly.

Karmic Purpose
To express creativity, life and love directly from your heart which empowers your soul and the soul of others.

Affirmation - 'I am filled with light and happiness.'

VIRGO   Good industrious work produces fine rewards

Ruler: Mercury   **Element:** Earth   **Mode:** Mutable

Personality Profile
Virgo by nature is practical, capable and discerning, and is known as the Analyst in the zodiac. You are eager to please and to serve others, either through career or daily activity. You are highly intelligent and possess a mind that researches information for the collective good. You organise well and usually prefer to be more in a supportive role, although if needed, you can lead and delegate well. You like to have a plan and make lists.

You also have an extraordinary ability to see details in life that other people just cannot see. This attribute can also make you very critical of yourself and others. This quality leaves no room for mistakes through which you can learn and grow from. You need to be softer on yourself. You're not perfect, although I know you think you need to be.

Affected Body Systems
- Upper Digestion
- Mental Nervous System
- Body parts affected include small intestines, pancreas, solar plexus, salivary glands, liver and bowels

Disease and Ailments
Ruled by Mercury, the planet of intellectual and internal body communications, you tend to exhaust your nerves and disrupt your digestion through excess worry and being over analytical.

Virgo rules the small intestines and your body's ability to absorb and assimilate nutrients. You are prone to disorders of the small intestines, pancreas, salivary glands and peristalsis.

Common ailments include diarrhoea, irritable bowel syndrome, mental nervous tension, hypoglycaemia, gastroenteritis, colic, appendicitis, peritonitis, constipation, migraines, food allergies and cravings.

The main cause of stress is your mind. You tend to obsess and excessively worry about your state of health (or others) when there is no need. You are usually very healthy, although your digestion will suffer if you worry too much.

As a Virgo, you do well by understanding what effect food has on you. With this understanding, you can make appropriate choices for your body and by doing so, you keep yourself healthy. You feel connected to the land, so it's only natural that freshly grown foods and herbs serve your body best. Your motto should be healthy mind maintains a healthy body.

> *The main cause of stress is your mind. ... You are usually very healthy, although your digestion will suffer if you worry too much.*

Nourishing Nutrition

Beneficial foods include: celery, apples, strawberries, lettuce, cucumber, melon, capsicum, lemons, kelp, walnuts, pecans, fish, nuts, seeds, whole grains, vegetable juices, berries, seaweed, brown rice and citrus. Avoid over indulgences in salt and rich foods so as not to throw out kidney balance; have adequate water during the day to keep kidneys flushed.

Foods containing essential vitamins suitable for Virgo:

B1: Pork, liver, heart, kidneys, fish, potatoes, nuts, pulses, rice bran, soy milk, rolled oats, lima beans, peas, lentils and mung beans.

B complex: Leafy green vegetables and green fruits.

Helpful Herbs

- Vervain for the central nervous system
- Dandelion and fenugreek to support the liver
- Fennel to help balance digestion
- Slippery elm and peppermint to soothe digestion
- Alfalfa to aid protein digestion.
- Brahmi an Ayurvedic herb, boosts memory and reduces mental fatigue

Activities to Minimise Stress
As your mind is constantly active, you need to learn to relax and calm your mind daily. A great practice for you is meditation, twenty minutes minimum. This practice will keep you focused, grounded and aligned with life. You love to exercise your brain; reading, crosswords and brain teasers suit you. Remember, you are trying to rest your mind, so limit these activities.

You need to have a regular schedule to keep you in shape. Exercise like yoga, tai chi, walking in nature, rock climbing, hiking, cricket, tennis, darts, snooker, and gymnastics are all beneficial. You respond well to regular cleansing or a detoxification diet and natural therapies.

Charity work soothes your soul and helps you to feel better about life.

Spiritual chakra Vishuddha
Virgo rules the throat, the fifth chakra. Virgos love to research, analyse, and categorize information so that they can then share and communicate with other people.

Signs of imbalance include speech impediments, sore throat, cough, neck problems, laryngitis, thyroid imbalance, respiratory and/or hearing problems and lies.

Therapeutic Treatments

Bach remedy: Centaury

Gives the ability to serve whoever they want, and not allow others to take you for granted. You will hold your own opinion and will receive as well as give in a healthy manner.

Signature Oil: Lavender

Lavender is one of the most used oils, renowned for its antibacterial, balancing, relaxing, stimulant, antipyretic, analgesic, antispasmodic and wound- healing properties.

Lavender can ease the tendency to worry, soothe achy muscles and promote restful sleep.

Vibration Colour: Earth Green

When feeling positive - harmonious, balanced, sharing, protective and secure.

When feeling negative - insincere, selfish, jealous, threatened, insecure.

Karmic Purpose
To be of service as an expression of the divine within you.

Affirmation – 'I am balanced, centred and secure in my emotions.'

LIBRA   Able to charm the birds from the trees

Ruler: Venus   **Element:** Air   **Mode:** Cardinal

Personality Profile

Libra is attracted to refined beauty in all things and is known as the Mediator in the zodiac. You are co-operative, diplomatic, idealistic, friendly, dependent, indecisive and self-sacrificial by nature. You seek to create harmony, balance and peace in life. This is important for your inner peace as this gives you joy and contentment.

You are very charming, stylish and polite. You also find these attributes attractive in others. You feel 'turned off' by people, language and environments that are repulsive. This disturbs your emotional balance and you need to leave the situation. You tend to be impartial; seeing both sides of every situation. Equality is important to you and seeing that there is justice for all gives you a sense of fairness.

As you are reflective by nature, you need time alone to assess and come to results that are valuable for you. If you feel pressured into decision making, you are prone to coming to a wrong conclusion.

Attracted by beauty and elegance, you may have superficial relationships with people. People are more than skin deep and you need to see past the surface and seek their soul to have meaningful connections.

Affected Body Systems
- Endocrine System balances hormones
- Body parts affected include adrenal glands, kidneys, urethras, inner ear, bladder, lower lumbar region and thyroid.

Disease and Ailments
Libra is ruled by Venus, the planet of balance. Its function is homeostasis in the body through the hormonal system and endocrine system.

Libra primarily rules the kidneys and keeps fluid regulation in balance. Common ailments include renal stones, thyroid problems, lower back pain, exhausted adrenal gland, bladder problems, dizziness, urinary tract infections, kidney disease, dizziness, high blood pressure and suppression of urine.

Being ruled by Venus, you love romantic dinners, fine dining and good wine. You also love sweet foods; rich chocolates are a favourite of yours.

In excess, this will cause blockages in the form of stones or clots. This will also lead to weight gain which damages your sense of self. You like to keep your youthful appearance and like to see yourself as beautiful. Why not? To do this, you need to be conscience of how you live your lifestyle. Libras need to drink copious amounts of water to keep their kidneys flushed and to maintain homeostasis.

> *Libras need to drink copious amounts of water to keep their kidneys flushed...*

Nourishing Nutrition
Beneficial foods include: celery, apples, strawberries, lettuce, cucumber, melon, capsicum, lemons, kelp, walnuts, pecans,

fish, nuts, seeds, whole grains, vegetable juices, berries, seaweed, brown rice and citrus. Avoid over indulgences in salt and rich foods so as not to throw out kidney balance and have adequate water during the day to keep kidneys flushed.

Foods containing essential vitamins suitable for Libra:

A: Liver, carrots, parsley, sweet potato, spinach, mangos, chives, tomatoes and broccoli.

B: Pork, liver, heart, kidneys, fish, potatoes, nuts, pulses, rice bran, soymilk, rolled oats, lima beans, peas, lentils and mung beans.

B3: Milk, yoghurt, eggs, meat, poultry and fish.

E: Vegetable oil, wheat germ, soybeans, whole grains, raw nuts, raw seeds and eggs

B complex: Leafy green vegetables and green fruits

C: Citrus fruits, red chilli peppers, kale, parsley, cauliflower, broccoli, turnip greens, sprouts, spinach, cabbage, mangos, oysters, lima beans, strawberries and raspberries.

Helpful Herbs

- Hops for anxiety.
- Kelp for hormonal balance.
- Celery for acid balance.
- Alfalfa is high in vitamin B and supports acid balance.
- Sarsaparilla for hormonal balance.
- Vitex Agnus Castus balances female hormones.
- Cranberry reduces burning on urination and urinary tract infections.

Minimising Stress

Libra is happy when all areas in life are in harmony with each other. This is a tall order and needs constant care to maintain this balance. Being aesthetic, you have a strong connection to music, beauty, fashion and the visual arts; they soothe your soul. Colour can be used effectively to soften and balance your living environment.

Fresh air, meditation, yoga, tai chi, being in relaxing environments and having stimulating interactions with others all serve you well. Exercises that benefit you include ice skating, badminton, cricket, ballroom dancing, gymnastics and swimming.

It is important that you hold your own power and do not devalue yourself for the sake of peace. As important as peace is to you, over compromising yourself will only lead to resentment and eventually, illness. Pamper yourself with massage and beauty treatments. Lymphatic drainage works well for you and be well hydrated drinking plenty of non-stimulating fluids, water, soups, juice and herbal teas.

Spiritual Chakra Anahata

Ruled by the heart, the fourth chakra and you are more concerned with co-operation, balance and mediation within relationships. By achieving this, love flows freely without always compromising yourself.

Signs of imbalance: all heart related diseases, high blood pressure, mistrust, holding onto past hurts, grief, co-dependency and unable to give and receive freely.

Therapeutic Treatments

Bach Remedy: Scleranthus
Promotes calmness and determination, improves the ability to make quick decisions, take swift action; also promotes a keen sense of fair play and keeps balance in all things.

Signature Oil: Geranium

Geranium's primary function is to balance, a key word for Librans. It acts as an antidepressant, aphrodisiac, hormone balancer, anti-inflammatory and insect repellent. Helps maintain calmness and equilibrium, with great benefits for beauty and female reproductive disorders.

Vibration Colour: Pink

When feeling positive - calming, soothing, increases confidence, affectionate, harmonious and loving.

When feeling negative - smothering, sickly, overwhelmed and stagnant.

Karmic Purpose
To develop a harmonious relationship with the self, so you can experience successful relationships with others.

Affirmation – 'I am full of confidence with an abundant of love for myself and others.'

SCORPIO — Getting to the root of all things

Ruler: Pluto   **Element:** Water   **Mode:** Fixed

Personality Profile

Scorpio is transformative in its orientation and is known as the Detective in the zodiac. You are known for being instinctual, empathetic, magnetic, powerful, possessive, manipulative and controlling. You are loyal, secretive, sexy and very emotional. You contain your emotions as you don't like to lose control. You are determined and resilient when it comes to achieving an outcome. Nothing will discourage you and this can lead to obsession if you are not careful. As a control freak, your biggest and hardest lesson is to let go when situations no longer serve you. Maybe your lesson is learnt? Do you really need to keep the suffering just to achieve the goal? The saying 'if you don't bend, you will break' really does apply to you. The only control you have in life is your perception and action connected to that. Be mindful that you are not here to be involved in power struggles. This is counterproductive. Power is supportive, not manipulative.

You are insightful by nature and have an uncanny ability to see right through people. You can see the cause and the solution in most cases. Ironically, you cannot always see the cause and solution in yourself. This usually comes to you after you have much pain, are reflective, and in hindsight.

This is a process of growth. So, the sooner you walk with the pain, the sooner you come to understand yourself. This then transforms you to the next level of consciousness and being.

Affected Body Systems
- Reproductive System
- Elimination System
- Body parts affected pituitary gland, bones of the pelvis, large intestine, rectum, bladder, kidney, groin, prostate gland, sweat glands, genitalia and the nose and ears.

Disease and Ailments
Ruled by Pluto, the planet of regeneration and the birth-death cycle, you tend to go into life with an all or nothing attitude. Scorpio is associated with the reproductive system and the eliminative process including the bowel, sweat glands, sphincter of the bladder, rectum and external genitalia.

Common ailments include constipation, piles, fistulas, haemorrhoids, stones, menstrual irregularities, hormonal disorders, womb disorders, seminal irregularities, prostate gland, sexually transmitted disease, colon disease, sluggish peristalsis and high blood pressure.

You have the ability to rise above the ashes as your sign, the Phoenix indicates. Your recuperative powers are strong and can overcome any illness you encounter. Suppression and accumulating negative emotions such as anger, resentment, guilt, suspicion and hatred will manifest as physical ailments. These include constipation, cancer and addiction. You are highly intuitive. Listen and trust what your body is trying to tell you and you will avoid many lifestyle illnesses. After all, you do know what is best for you ... live wisely.

> *Suppression and accumulating negative emotion such as anger, resentment, guilt, suspicion and hatred will manifest as physical ailments.*

Nourishing Nutrition

Beneficial foods include: fresh fruit and vegetables, oranges, lemon, apple cider vinegar, kelp, garlic, prunes, onions, beetroot, molasses, grapefruit, whole grains, nuts, wheat germ, oats, brown rice, figs, apples, cherries, plums, gooseberries, rhubarb and water. Avoid fermented and mucus forming foods, heating and stimulating foods, meat and salty foods. You will benefit well from fasting or using elimination diets at regular intervals

Foods containing essential vitamins suitable for Scorpio:

Complex B: Leafy green vegetables and green fruits.

C: Citrus fruits, red chilli peppers, kale, parsley, cauliflower, broccoli, turnip greens, sprouts, spinach, cabbage, mangos, oysters, lima beans, strawberries and raspberries.

E: Vegetable oil, wheat germ, soybeans, whole grains, raw nuts, raw seeds and eggs.

Folic acid: Chicken and beef livers, asparagus, lettuce, broccoli, fresh orange juice, legumes and dark leafy green vegetables.

Helpful Herbs

- Valerian: calming and supports the nerves and bowel.
- Yellow dock and calendula for lymphatics and detoxification.
- Aloe Vera and Senna as laxatives for constipation.
- Dong Quai, pennyroyal, raspberry leaf to support the reproductive system.
- Nettle root and Saw Palmetto supports the prostate.
- Wormwood clears parasites from the bowel.

Minimising Stress

As a Scorpio, you approach life's challenges with natural intensity and an investigative mind. You need to get to the bottom of things, and once achieved, this gives you a sense of peace. You actually enjoy this process, although it appears stressful to others looking on.

As you are competitive with others and with yourself, the following sports and exercises serve you best: yoga, shooting, fencing, swimming, scuba diving, fishing, running, canoeing, weight-lifting, martial arts and boxing. Sex is also a great outlet and if you are not having sex, then sports needs to be a primary focus in your life, so you channel your high energy levels. Remember here, sex is not competitive.

Music and the arts are nurturing for you and you can really allow your emotions to become one with what you experience and feel relaxed. You are often drawn to metaphysics, the occult and the study of the mind.

Living or being exposed to the ocean soothes your soul. Learn to laugh more as this promotes your immunity. Colonic therapies on a regular basis suit your constitution well (seek medical advice before commencement).

Spiritual Chakra Manipura

Scorpios are also linked to the third chakra, situated in the solar plexus, but unlike Aries, Scorpios tend to have issues with power struggles and understanding power, usually through sexual, financial, physical, emotional or mental abuse. Their role is to transcend the lesson and assimilate the knowledge to empower the self. Once you have achieved self-actualisation and transmutation, this is the gift you share with others to help them realise and reach their own personal power.

Therapeutic Treatments

Bach Remedy: Chicory

Promotes generosity and selflessness with others, while allowing individuals to live their own life independently.

Signature Oil: Patchouli

Patchouli is primarily an aphrodisiac, decongestant, antidepressant, regenerative and antiseptic. Powerfully potent, in South East Asia, this oil used to treat snake bites and poisonous insects. Hence the healing effect of this oil.

Vibration Colour: Maroon

When positive - compassionate, loving, genuine, mature, supportive.

When negative - unkind, selfish, artificial, stubborn and unhelpful.

Karmic Purpose

To understand and transcend your own painful process so you may have the insight to enable others with their process of life.

Affirmation – 'I am centred in my own personal power and respect the personal power of others.'

SAGITTARIUS — Shooting for the truth

Ruler: Jupiter   **Element:** Fire   **Mode:** Mutable

Personality Profile

Sagittarius is action oriented and is known as the Philosopher in the zodiac. You tend to live life to the fullest and will go to extremes to achieve your goal. You are optimistic, enthusiastic, honest, inspirational and outspoken. You are self-motivated and attain immense joy in going forward in life and achieving your life goals. You live as though there is no tomorrow. You are always positive and believe in the best in life; you go through life experiencing little or no fear.

Being adventurous and freedom loving, you love to travel and learn about all things to do with culture and its people. Seeking and living your universal truth is important to you. Spirituality and religion are areas of life that attract your mind. Please be mindful that we all seek spirituality in our own way, so be non-judgmental toward others' beliefs. This is not only considerate, but also respectful. You can come across to others as a 'know it all' and appear arrogant.

Remember, life is a process of ongoing learning for spiritual and creative growth. Please consider we don't all aspire to learn as much or as fast as you do. People learn in their own time, not in your time.

Affected Body Systems
- Motor Nervous System.
- Autonomic Nervous System.
- Body parts affected include liver, pancreas, spleen, hips, thighs, legs, buttocks, pelvis, pelvic muscles, sacrum, sacral spine and sciatic nerve.

Disease and Ailments

Ruled by Jupiter, the planet of expansion and extravagance, you tend to overindulge in food and wine which leads to stress on the liver and excess weight on the thighs. Sagittarius primarily rules the liver, thighs and hips. Common ailments include sciatica, rheumatism, hip joint dislocation, falls, stings, and kicks from animals, hepatitis, liver congestion, diabetes, pelvic problems, gout, nervous system disorders and falls, especially from horseback.

You have a strong constitution but do need regular exercise to keep trim. Sagittarius needs mental and physical freedom to maintain good health.

Overindulgence in food, alcohol, gambling, sex and exercise can cause ill health in middle age. Moderation in fats and alcohol is advisable to maintain a functioning liver. Balancing meat with vegetables works well for you. An excess in meat can contribute to high blood pressure.

> *Sagittarius needs mental and physical freedom to maintain*

Nourishing Nutrition

Beneficial foods include mushrooms, whole grains, oats, brewer's yeast, whole eggs, wheat germ and shellfish, apples including skin, alfalfa, kelp, rye, figs, rice, cucumber, berries, prunes and cherries, lettuce, corn, endive, chicory, parsnips, onions, asparagus, horseradish and lean meat. Avoid overindulging, acid forming foods, overexertion physically and mentally.

Foods containing essential vitamins suitable for Sagittarius:

B6: Lean meat, poultry, fish, eggs, whole wheat breads and cereals, nuts, bananas, soybeans, brown rice, lentils, lima beans, avocados, spinach, potatoes, cauliflower, popcorn and leeks.

C: Citrus fruits, red chilli peppers, kale, parsley, cauliflower, broccoli, turnip greens, sprouts, spinach, cabbage, mangos, oysters, lima beans, strawberries and raspberries.

Helpful Herbs

- Burdock as a blood cleanser
- Celery for arthritis especially in the hips
- Dandelion to support the liver
- Oats nourishes the central nervous system
- Turmeric is a liver tonic
- Milk thistle protects and repairs liver cells

Minimising Stress

Sagittarians are freedom seekers and love being outdoors. As a fire sign, you are very active and restless. For you, activity is a means of reducing stress. Suitable sports to channel your energy include horse riding, polo, skiing, archery, bike riding, shooting, hockey, football, basketball and running.

Your mind can be as active as your body and you enjoy exploring the deeper meaning to life through philosophy, reading and higher learning. Meditation and deep breathing exercises like Tai Chi and Yoga benefit you. You tend to live life in extremes. Having regular gallbladder and liver detoxification helps to rejuvenate your body (seek medical advice before commencement).

Spiritual Chakra Svadhisthana

Linked to the second chakra in the sacral area, this is primarily concerned with expansion, creative expression and pleasure, emotional and sexual balance within relationships.

Signs of imbalance are lower back pain, reproductive complaints, bladder, kidney troubles, imbalanced sex drive, guilt, feelings of isolation and emotional instability.

Therapeutic Treatments

Bach Remedy: Agrimony

Will bring an about a more positive attitude, with renewed faith and hope in your life.

Signature Oil: Black Pepper

Black Pepper is fiery oil, it stimulates, tones muscles, and is carminative. This oil gets straight to the root and will relieve a tired mind or painful stiff muscles.

Vibration Colour: Blue

When positive - calm, tranquil, honest, accepting, reassuring and peaceful.

When negative - depressed, withdrawn, distrusting, inflexible, isolated.

Karmic Purpose
To understand your truth and live without inflicting your belief system onto others.

Affirmation - 'I am attaining more peace and tranquillity in my life.'

CAPRICORN   If at first you don't succeed, try, try again

Ruler: Saturn   **Element:** Earth   **Mode:** Cardinal

Personality Profile

Capricorn has a keen sense of responsibility and is known as the Wiseman in the zodiac. This wisdom is present in childhood and you are often told you appear older than your actually age.

You are ambitious, focused and hardworking, often achieving goals you set for yourself. You are very reliable and moral and will keep your word with others. Being self-disciplined, practical, sensible, patient and cautious, you often assess situations carefully before making decisions. You will strive to be an authority in whatever field you specialise in. This gives you respect and recognition. You also respect others in positions of authority. Your sense of duty is strong, especially if you are a parent. You will often do whatever it takes to make sure you and your family are financially secure. As admirable as this is, it often takes you away from all the things in life that give you joy. You are often seen as emotionally distant. You need to feel totally secure in a relationship before you can commit and express yourself emotionally. So, in relationships you need to take your time and explain this to your partner.

Affected Body Systems
- Skeletal System
- Body parts affected skin, bones, body joints, knees, hair, nails, teeth, gallbladder, and parathyroid gland.

Disease and Ailments

Ruled by Saturn, the planet of structure and stability, this governs all support systems in the body. Capricorn rules the skeletal system, joints, knees, skin, hair, nails, teeth, parathyroid gland, and gallbladder. Common ailments include skin disorders like psoriasis and eczema.

Arthritis, rheumatism, gout, knee complaints, gallstones, constipation, poor circulation and disorders to bone and teeth are common also.

In childhood, you are often prone to illness. As your body matures, you become stronger and healthier, looking younger than your peers. As disease is rare for you except in old age, you must tend to illness as soon as it manifests, otherwise there is a tendency for the illness to be chronic if left untreated. You are prone to dryness and need oil in your diet with considerable amounts of water to prevent dehydration, even in winter.

> *...you must tend to illness as soon as it manifests, otherwise there is a tendency for the illness to be chronic...*

Serious by nature you are susceptible to depression. Get out of your head and into your hands. Do something that's fun and get some sunshine and stop wearing black as this promotes depression.

Nourishing Nutrition
Beneficial foods include, sardines, salmon, egg yolk, shellfish, nuts, sesame seeds, green leafy vegetables, asparagus, lentils, eggs, molasses, carob, legumes, essential fatty acids, nuts and seeds, figs, blueberries, plums, cheese, coconut, raisins, leeks, oily fish and linseed (flaxseed) oil, kelp and dairy products. Heating, stimulating foods as well as foods that are well cooked are best absorbed. Avoid meat and acid forming foods.

Foods containing essential vitamins suitable for Capricorn:

A: Liver, carrots, parsley, sweet potato, spinach, mangos, chives, tomatoes and broccoli.

C: Citrus fruits, red chilli peppers, kale, parsley, cauliflower, broccoli, turnip greens, sprouts, spinach, cabbage, mangos, oysters, lima beans, strawberries and raspberries.

K: Broccoli, cabbage and sprouts.

Bioflavonoid: Fresh vegetables, green peppers, grapes, apricots, strawberries, cherries, prunes and blackcurrants

Helpful Herbs

- Comfrey for bone repair
- Willows bark, Boswellia and Devils claw are all-natural anti-inflammatory and pain relievers.
- St John's Wort soothes the nervous system and helps with mild depression *(do NOT use if on antidepressants)*.
- Heartsease soothes the skin that has eczema.
- Glucosamine and Chondroitin nourishes the joints improving movement.

Minimising Stress
Capricorns are very serious by nature and you need to laugh and have more fun. Both of these things improve your immunity. A dose of fifteen minutes daily sunshine improves your skin and sense of wellbeing. Regular exercise like mountain climbing, yoga, gardening, golf, cricket, skiing, running and snooker improves your circulation. You are ambitious, so setting goals and achieving them gives you a strong sense of self. Remember not everything in life has to be difficult in order to be a success, so go with the flow sometimes. You do like to be alone and can

often sit and read as a form of relaxation. Listening to music or singing will also soothe you. If feeling dark and down on yourself, avoid black and dark colours as they sap your energy. Wear soothing greens and earth tones or motivating colours of oranges, and yellows. Psychotherapy, chiropractic, oil massage and osteopathy are beneficial therapies for you.

Spiritual Chakra Muladhara

Capricorns are ambitious and by nature work very hard, so it's natural that they are linked to the first chakra found in the base of the spine. The lessons are with creating foundations for life, survival, security, providing for physical needs, grounding, health and standing up for what you believe in.

Signs of imbalance include constipation, obesity, leg, knee problems, osteoarthritis, incapable of being still and fear.

Therapeutic Treatments

Bach Remedy: Mimulus.

Will can face fear with faith, believing all will be well.

Signature Oil: Vetivert

Vetivert, known as the 'oil of tranquillity', aids your worrisome mind. It is grounding, antiseptic, relaxant, a woman's hormone balancer, an aphrodisiac, and regenerative. Works well on rheumatic and arthritic joint pain which Capricornia's know only too well.

Vibration Colour: Black

When positive - power, authority, respectable, sexy, strength.

When negative - depressed, death, rebellious, grief, withdrawn.

Karmic Purpose
To develop your inner authority, to share and express this wisdom for mankind.

Affirmation – 'I am feeling stronger and more powerful every day.'

AQUARIUS — I did it my way

Ruler: Uranus   **Element:** Air   **Mode:** Fixed

Personality Profile

Aquarius is intellectually oriented and is known as the Innovator in the zodiac. Your desire is to be unique and to be accepted for the original individual you are. You have a quick rational inventive mind, are impulsive, love variety with change and are intuitive with a strong imagination. Although you are friendly, you possess a strong sense of wanting to help humanity and are often seen as cool and aloof by others. This is because you have an ability to be objective and detached in situations where most people are emotional. It's not that you are not emotional, it's just that you're not *overly* emotional and you tend to think your feelings. Expressing your feelings is not easy for you and you tend to get stuck in your head. Write poetry or a love letter to channel what you feel and then maybe give it to your partner. People express love differently, so this may work for you.

When you come to evaluating a problem, it is thought out logically before it's delivered. You have a very independent nature and this needs expression in all areas of your life.

Affected Body Systems
- Circulatory System
- Body parts affected hypothalamus, parathyroid, eyes, ankles, legs, nervous system, the meridian system, the chakras and spinal cord.

Disease and Ailments

Ruled by Uranus, the planet of electrical connections, you are prone to nervous and circulatory conditions. Aquarius rules the calves, ankles, legs, circulation, and energy flow in the body, the eyes, and spinal cord. Common ailments include poor circulation, cold hands and feet, blood disorders, lower leg cramping, varicose veins, sprained and swollen ankles, spinal curvature, nerve degeneration, weak eyesight, anaemia, and nervous disease.

Aquarius has a strong body constitution and you are usually healthy in life. When you are unwell, you will recuperate quickly.

Your main stress is your mind. When you are mentally stressed or worried, your nerves are the first to suffer. Plan your mental activities so you do not overtax your mind. You have irregular eating patterns which contribute to the highs and lows you experience through the day. Having planned regular snacks and meals every four hours will compensate for this.

> *Your main stress is your mind. When you are mentally stressed or worried your nerves are the first to suffer.*

Nourishing Nutrition

Beneficial foods include: ginger, onion, garlic, spices and warming foods; nerve relaxants such as essential fatty acids, nuts, seeds, fish, brewer's yeast, wheat germ, spinach, asparagus, radishes, lentils, celery, root veggies, cheese, broccoli, apricots, apples, figs, almonds, peaches, eggs, corn, lecithin, berries and leafy green vegetables. Avoid large amounts of salt.

Foods containing essential vitamins suitable for Aquarius:

A: Liver, carrots, parsley, sweet potato, spinach, mangos, chives, tomatoes and broccoli.

B complex: Leafy green vegetables and green fruit.

C: Citrus fruits, red chilli peppers, kale, parsley, cauliflower, broccoli, turnip greens, sprouts, spinach, cabbage, mangos, oysters, lima beans, strawberries and raspberries.

E: Vegetable oil, wheat germ, soybeans, whole grains, raw nuts, raw seeds and eggs.

PABA: Whole grains, eggs, milk, liver, yoghurt and molasses.

Helpful Herbs

- Rue and Mugwort for varicose veins.
- Brahmi improves memory and a nervous system tonic.
- Garlic and Echinacea which increases immunity.
- St. John's Wort supports the nerves (*do NOT use with antidepressants*).
- Silica to insulate the nerves. (do NOT use if you have metal implants inside your body)
- Ginkgo enhances blood circulation.

Minimising Stress

Aquarius is very intellectual and likes spending time alone. You will often spend time reading or surfing the net to relax. Other people often see this as work and do not realise that this is how you unwind. Activities like chess, bridge, crosswords and Sudoku that involve strategy of the mind often attract you. You enjoy affiliating with computer and technology groups.

Having an inventive mind, you often like to dabble with electrical gadgets and technology. Space: the final frontier - this is another dimension you like to get absorbed and lost in. You do like music and dancing, but it's usually to your own unique taste. When you choose to get physical, sports that benefit are flying, parachuting, hang-gliding, badminton, skiing, ice skating and cycling. You love being free and nature gives you space and no limitations. Being in nature soothes your mind and keeps you grounded, especially if you are working the land or are with animals. It is important to you that you live your unique lifestyle to be happy. Add a water feature to your home environment to soothe your nerves and help you connect to your emotions.

Beneficial therapies include meditation, acupuncture, homeopathy and energy healing.

Spiritual Chakra Muladhara

Linked to the first chakra, found in the base of the spine, the lessons are with creating foundations, survival, security, providing for physical needs, grounding, health and standing up for yourself. As Aquarians love their freedom, they frequently have a dilemma with being responsible in daily life and being free to be who they want to be. The secret is to have a life which can honour both happily.

Signs of imbalance include constipation, obesity, leg and knee problems, osteoarthritis, lower leg circulatory problems, incapable of being still and fear.

Therapeutic Therapies

Bach Remedy: Water Violet

Promotes your inner peace and harmony, so then they can extend peace and harmony to others.

Signature Oil: Neroli

Neroli oil is an aphrodisiac, antidepressant, calmative, meditative, antispasmodic and antiseptic. Works well on your mind giving you confidence and strength. This is great in the treatment of insomnia.

Vibration Colour: Purple

When positive - intuitive, dignified, valuable, revealed, open-minded.

When negative - hidden, humble, unworthy, alone, narrow-minded.

Karmic Purpose
To be safe and secure in your own innovative ideas so you can benefit humanity.

Affirmation – 'I deserve acknowledgement, recognition and respect from others.'

PISCES — A good heart is hard to find

Ruler: Neptune   **Element:** Water   **Mode:** Mutable

Personality Profile

Pisces is very sensitive, is spiritually oriented and is known as the Medium in the zodiac. Considerate, caring, compassionate and empathic by nature, you are often drawn to people and careers involved in healing. You are also very emotional, receptive and intuitive, and often tune into another's misery easily. You need to be careful as you are so sensitive, you may absorb other people's problems and take them on as your own. This can only lead to illness and a depletion of your energy levels. When in this state you may feel ungrounded, confused, delusional, introverted, moody and victimised. So, examine what you are feeling and determine if it's yours or whether you are you carrying someone else's pain.

You have a powerful urge of wanting to become 'one' with another. Be mindful, this can lead to co-dependency and addictions if you look to be completed by another. Learn to be one with yourself and connect to your spirit. You can go into the world and meet people as an equal without having to take on the role of care giver.

Affected Body Systems
- Lymphatic System
- Immune System
- Body parts affected: feet, toes, immune system, body fluids, spinal fluid, lymphatic system, pineal gland, plasma and blood.

Disease and Ailments

Ruled by Neptune, the planet of receptivity and sensitivity, this connects to all the fluids within your body. Pisces rules the immune and lymphatic system, feet, toes, pineal gland, body fluids and blood. Common ailments include swollen lymph glands, colds, flu, fatigue, alcoholism, weak lungs, foot problems, poor circulation, fluid retention, gout, viral and bacterial infections, immune infections, autoimmune disorders and mucosal discharges. Having a sensitive body, you are prone easily to allergies, so you need to be cautious with medications and certain foods. You should not take toxic substances of any kind, as your body is not designed to deal with the toxins and therefore, you may become addicted.

Pisces have a weak constitution and you are often very sensitive to your surroundings (including people). As a result, you often attract illness. Sometimes the real world is too harsh for your delicate nature and often you look for escapism through addictive substances. Seek counselling and channel your dreamy escapism through art and spirituality. Connect to nature and stay grounded. You need strong clear boundaries with yourself and others with vigilant self-care to maintain health.

> *You need strong clear boundaries with yourself and others with vigilant self-care to maintain health.*

Nourishing Nutrition

Beneficial foods include: ginger, onion, berries, beans, dates, figs, spinach, citrus fruit, green leafy veggies, parsley, raisins, spinach, nuts, almonds, molasses, legumes, egg yolk, kelp, pumpkin seeds, wheat germ, tomato, apricots and peaches, water, vegetable juice, herbal teas, soup, a little freshly squeezed fruit juice is ok. Avoid stimulants, alcohol, drugs and overeating.

Foods containing essential vitamins suitable for Pisces:

A: Liver, carrots, parsley, sweet potato, spinach, mangos, chives, tomatoes and broccoli.

B complex: Leafy green vegetables and green fruit.

C: Citrus fruits, red chilli peppers, kale, celery, parsley, cauliflower, broccoli, turnip greens, sprouts, spinach, cabbage, mangos, oysters, lima beans, strawberries and raspberries.

D: Fish liver oils, tuna, salmon, sardines, seaweeds and dairy.

Helpful Herbs

- Echinacea to support the immune system.
- Garlic, a natural antimicrobial.
- Astragalus, an immune stimulant.
- Bilberry, an antioxidant herb.
- Chamomile calms nerves.
- Dandelion to release accumulated fluid in the body.

Minimising Stress
Pisces is very sensitive, and the arts suit you well when it comes to relaxation. They include writing poetry, painting, sad movies, listening to music and nature, photography, sculpture and dance. Your home environment and surroundings need to be serene to soothe your receptive nature. Having a flowing water feature in the home also helps as water and rain soothe your soul. Being grounded is also important for you, so have strong feminine wood furniture in your home to help achieve this. Mediation in a peaceful place calms your mind and connects you to spirit. You love spas and all water sports like surfing,

swimming, diving, rowing, rafting and fishing. Gymnastics, ice skating, yoga and dancing also work well for you. Avoid dark blue and black as they promote depression. Wear more greens, yellows and earth colours. Therapies that benefit you include foot reflexology, float tanks, anything mystic, homeopathy, and lymphatic drainage.

Spiritual Chakra Svadhisthana
Correlates to the second chakra in the sacral area, this is primarily concerned with linking you to your creative side intuitionally with wisdom. Due to their sensitive natures, intimate contact with these people should be sacred as they seek union on a spiritual level and have problems with boundaries.

Signs of imbalance: lower back pain, reproductive complaints, bladder, kidney troubles, unbalanced sex drive, guilt, feelings of isolation and emotional instability.

Therapeutic Treatments

Bach Remedy: Rock rose

Will access your inner strength enabling you to work through fear and trauma with courage

Signature Oil: Melissa

Melissa oil is an antidepressant, antiseptic, meditative, calmative and stimulant. Will bring about a peaceful state, encouraging strength and revitalization.

Vibration Colour: Turquoise

When positive - refreshing, clear, youthful, sensitive, and transformational.

When negative - confused, unimaginative, uncertain, disturbed, dull.

Karmic Purpose
To achieve connection through the spiritual/artistic senses, to connect to your higher self and divine wholeness.

Affirmation – 'I am becoming more creative, imaginative and transformational.'

Personal Notes

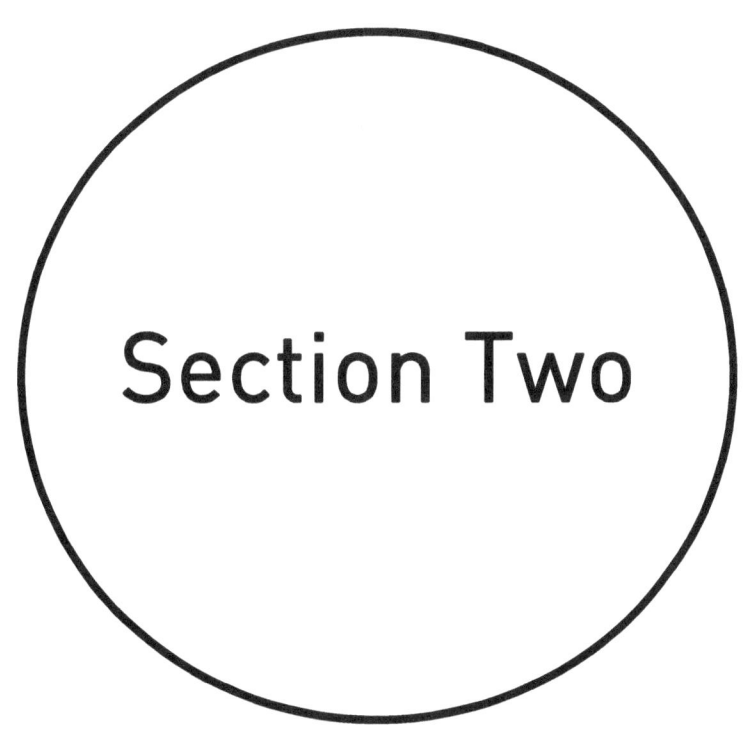

Simply Ayurveda

"The wealth of a nation is improved when there is investment in the health of its citizens." Professor Dr. P.H. Kulkarni, Founder and Director Ayurveda Academy, Pune, India.

Ayurveda is the science of healing based on time-tested principles of nature that originated around 5,000 years ago in India. Its origin is in the ancient text of wisdom known as the 'Vedas'. Vedas are the 'life wisdom' scrolls complied over thousands of years by ancient scientists called 'Rishis'. The Rishis took it upon themselves to preserve this knowledge and pass it on only to those who would honour its traditions, origin and information.

Ayurveda is composed of two words – *Ayur* means life and *Veda* means knowledge. Hence why Ayurveda is commonly termed as 'The Science of Life' or 'The Art of Right Living'. The word of Ayurveda has now been communicated from India to China (Ayurveda laid the foundation for Chinese medicine).

As early as 1924, there was an article in The Lancet (U.S.A.) providing an interesting insight into Western attitudes toward Ayurveda by an anonymous author. In 1959, Maharishi Mahesh Yogi went to the United States to spread the word of Transcendental Meditation. In the 1970s and 80s, Ayurveda came into the public eye through the New Age movement that was emerging at that time, particularly through the efforts of Maharishi Mahesh Yogi, Robert Svoboda, Vasant Lad, David Frawley and Deepak Chopra.

Everyone has a unique genetic map that holds the secrets of what is more suitable and what is less appropriate to them in various life events. When they understand their makeup and live a life accordingly they enjoy health. This is the concept behind healthy living, according to Ayurveda.

> ...Ayurveda deals with the diseased person and not solely with the disease...

Any imbalance in this will bring disconnection to our mind-body. Ayurveda knows that body and mind are interlinked. Wisdom created mind, mind created body and they mutually reflect and feed each other.

Everything in this universe is a unique combination of subtle elements (or forces) of nature. These elements within us all determine the life process of growth and decay. To maintain health, the body needs to be in alignment with constitutional and environmental elements.

Ayurveda explains disease as the unbalanced state of dhatus (tissues), Doshas (biological elements) and malas (body excretions) within the person, affecting mind and body. Ayurveda deals with the diseased person and not solely with the disease. Doing so promotes more of a holistic view to treatment.

Ayurveda healing focuses on 3 areas:

- to preserve health
- to promote the health of the healthy person
- to cure the disease of the patient.

Treatment involves taking the right action and responsibility around living a fulfilling lifestyle in correlation to your personal priority of needs. When this is interfered with, you become imbalanced and your health will start to suffer. When our body is misaligned with our constitution, we start experiencing discomfort like a car that uses different sized wheels. Usually, this is the result of stress or unwholesome aspects of food or lifestyle. Healing may involve an improved, more fulfilling and empowering lifestyle.

Ayurveda incorporates a combination of healthy routines specific to your individuality that include nutrition, diet, spices, massage, body therapies, cleanses, tonics, herbs, music, dance, Rasayana (rejuvenation therapy), colour, Vastu Shastra (science of structures), astrology, exercise, gem therapy, aromatherapy and a religious/spiritual philosophy or practice that works for you.

Ayurveda is a complete, holistic system that respects all aspects of existence - soul, mind and body. It always incorporates simple, powerful and practical techniques personalised for everyone.

There are three primary life-forces that act within the body known as the Tridoshas. They are Vata, Pitta, and Kapha. They also can be translated as energies, biological principles and functional units. The Doshas are a combination of the five elements: ether, air, fire, water and earth. They are movable elements within us all that determine the life process of growth and decay. To maintain homeostasis, the Doshas must be in balance within the body.

As mentioned previously, our physical constitution is made up of the elements in nature at the time of conception. Let's consider the constitutions (or body types).

The three main constitutions are Vata, Pitta and Kapha.

Vata
Elements: Air and Ether

Vata or Air people are structurally light and slim. They are physically and mentally very active, requiring (and thrive on) constant stimulation and variety to be satisfied. Often drawn to the creative fields, they have pioneering vision and unparalleled initiation, but rarely have the discipline to finish what they start. They have difficulty in maintaining healthy habits as they are impatient and inconsistent with themselves and others.

> ...they are natural in 'going with the flow' in all aspects of life...

They are natural in 'going with the flow' in all aspects of life. They are designed to move on like a feather in the wind - always enthusiastic, always in motion, always unpredictable. They possess an alert, adaptable and clever mind.

Vata people respond well to pastels in the shades of pink, orange, yellow, green, white and gold. These colours are warming in nature and help calm the nervous system, whilst feeding their gentle and light mind-set. Natural colours like brown and tan will help with grounding. Avoid excess of blues as this will cause overstimulation of the mind and nervous system, and dark blues, greys and black as this will promote depression.

In balance: vibrant, enthusiastic, alert, energetic and clear thinking.

Unbalanced: irritable, fearful, restless, negative thoughts, insecure, anxious and ungrounded.

Gemstones which help pacify and balance include emerald, jade, yellow sapphire, topaz, or citrine - set in gold.

Aroma essences which ground and soothe the mind include sandalwood, lotus, cinnamon, basil and frankincense.

Body rulership: governs all movements within the body. This includes breathing, circulation, elimination of wastes and flow of nerve impulses to and from the brain.

Organ rulership: primarily the colon, followed by the brain, kidneys, bladder, bones, bone marrow, nervous system, spinal cord, muscle contraction and chest.

Pitta
Elements: Fire and Water

Pitta or Fire people are structurally muscular and angular. They are naturally analytical, precise and endowed with leadership qualities. They are often drawn to challenging careers as they perform well under pressure. They love to stick with a set program or schedule. Their strong emphasis on the goal can make them extremist. In short, they are naturally analytical, clear, precise, forceful, intense, challenge-loving and result-oriented.

In balance: intellectual, warm, loving, enjoys challenges, digests and assimilates all nutrients well, goal seeking and sharp memory.

Unbalanced: critical, angry, demanding, argumentative, impatient, frustrated and irritable.

Pitta people respond well to pastels in blues, greens, white and purples as this will cool their fiery personality. The colour silver is also cooling and fire types benefit from moonlight walks

> ...they are naturally analytical, precise and endowed with leadership qualities...

or swims. Avoid excess of reds, yellows and orange as this will fuel anger and undisciplined aggression easily, especially in summer.

Gemstones which help pacify and soothe include emerald, jade, peridot, and moonstone, pearl, amethyst or blue sapphire set in silver.

Aroma essences that cool and calm the mind include rose, lotus, sandalwood and jasmine.

Body rulership: all digestion and metabolism e.g. processing and assimilating of all foods and nutrients throughout the body.

Organ rulership: primarily the small intestines followed by blood, liver, spleen, heart, endocrine, digestion tract, gallbladder, skin and eyes.

Kapha
Elements: Earth and Water

Kapha or Water people are structurally solid and curvaceous. Security conscience, they often save money well and spend on essential comforts or invest in properties. They are nurturing and caring by nature and are drawn to the caring, hospitality and culinary fields. They are accommodating and listen with acceptance. They are very parental in nature, extremely sensitive and gentle. They always put others ahead of themselves.

Kapha people respond well to bright and bold reds, orange, yellow and gold as they are stimulating and warming, helping the person to be motivated in daily life. Avoid blue, green, white and pastels as they are calming and can instil inertia. Brown is good to wear if you feel overwhelmed, scattered or ungrounded.

> ...they are nurturing and caring by nature...

In balance: forgiving, relaxed, methodical, pleasant, reliable, calm, loyal, conservative, romantic and confident.

Unbalanced: depressed, lethargic, stubborn, shy, sensitive, dependent and passive.

Gemstones which motivate the mind include cats eye, ruby, garnet and lapis set in gold. Amethyst may be used to calm and clear the mind for creative or spiritual activities.

Aroma essences that inspire and quiet the mind include frankincense, cloves, cinnamon, cedar, myrrh and musk.

Body rulership: all body structure and cohesiveness within the body.

Organ rulership: primarily the stomach and lungs followed by pancreas, joints, lymphatic system, C.S.F. fluid, synovial fluid, pleura fluid, saliva, tongue and digestion fluids.

Though we carry all these elements within us, we might have a predominance of one or two elements. This can be determined by completing a Dosha questionnaire.

Mini Dosha Test

To determine your Ayurvedic Dosha, fill out the questionnaire below. Base your choices on what you observe is most consistent over an extended period, rather than your present state. Make one choice from the column that best describes yourself. However, feel free to make a selection from more than one column if two columns equally describe you. All the words in that column need not apply for you make the selection. For example, see below: Column Vata, Observation Hair - "dry, brittle and scarce". If one of these applies, make the selection.

After finishing the questionnaire, add up your scores for each of the Doshas. Alternatively, go online to the link provided below, complete the online questionnaire, press the 'calculate results' (located left of the page) button to discover your Doshas. If you make a mistake, just click the box again to de-select. Or if you would like to try again, press the erase & start over button (located left of the page). Most of us will have one Dosha predominant, a few will have two Doshas approximately equal and even fewer will have all three Doshas in equal proportion.

Guidelines for Determining Your Constitution

Instructions: To determine your constitution it is best to fill out the chart twice. First, base your choices on what is most consistent over a long period of your life (your prakruti), then fill it out a second time responding to how you have been feeling more recently (your vikruti). Sometimes it helps to have a friend ask you the questions and fill in the chart for you, as they may have insight (and impartiality) to offer. After finishing the chart each time, add up the number of marks under vata, pitta and kapha.

This will help you discover your own ratio of doshas in your prakruti and vikruti. Most people will have one dosha predominant, a few will have two doshas approximately equal and even fewer will have all three doshas in equal proportion. For instance, if your vikruti shows more pitta than your prakruti, you will want to follow a pitta-soothing regimen to try and bring your vikruti back into balance with your prakruti. If your prakruti and vikruti seem about the same, then you would choose the regimen of your strongest dosha.

Copyright ©1994, 2016. Excerpted from *Ayurvedic Cooking for Self-Healing* by Usha and Dr. Lad. All Rights Reserved.

OBSERVATIONS	V	P	K	VATA	PITTA	KAPHA
Body size	☐	☐	☐	Slim	Medium	Large
Body weight	☐	☐	☐	Low	Medium	Overweight
Chin	☐	☐	☐	Thin, angular	Tapering	Rounded, double
Cheeks	☐	☐	☐	Wrinkled, sunken	Smooth flat	Rounded, plump
Eyes	☐	☐	☐	Small, sunken, dry, active, black, brown, nervous	Sharp, bright, gray, green, yellow/red, sensitive to light	Big, beautiful, blue, calm, loving
Nose	☐	☐	☐	Uneven shape, deviated septum	Long pointed, red nose-tip	Short rounded, button nose
Lips	☐	☐	☐	Dry, cracked, black/brown tinge	Red, inflamed, yellowish	Smooth, oily, pale, whitish
Teeth	☐	☐	☐	Stick out, big, roomy, thin gums	Medium, soft, tender gums	Healthy, white, strong gums
Skin	☐	☐	☐	Thin, dry, cold, rough, dark	Smooth, oily, warm, rosy	Thick, oily, cool, white, pale
Hair	☐	☐	☐	Dry brown, black, knotted, brittle, scarce	Straight, oily, blond, gray, red, bald	Thick, curly, oily, wavy, luxuriant
Nails	☐	☐	☐	Dry, rough, brittle, break easily	Sharp, flexible, pink, lustrous	Thick, oily, smooth, polished
Neck	☐	☐	☐	Thin, tall	Medium	Big, folded
Chest	☐	☐	☐	Flat, sunken	Moderate	Expanded, round
Belly	☐	☐	☐	Thin, flat, sunken	Moderate	Big, pot-bellied
Belly-button	☐	☐	☐	Small, irregular, herniated	Oval, superficial	Big, deep, round, stretched
Hips	☐	☐	☐	Slender, thin	Moderate	Heavy, big
Joints	☐	☐	☐	Cold, cracking	Moderate	Large, lubricated
Appetite	☐	☐	☐	Irregular, scanty	Strong, unbearable	Slow but steady
Digestion	☐	☐	☐	Irregular, forms gas	Quick, causes burning	Prolonged, forms mucous
Taste	☐	☐	☐	Sweet, sour, salty	Sweet, bitter, astringent	Bitter, pungent, astringent
Thirst	☐	☐	☐	Changeable	Surplus	Sparse
Elimination	☐	☐	☐	Constipation	Loose	Thick, oily, sluggish
Physical Activity	☐	☐	☐	Hyperactive	Moderate	Slow
Mental Activity	☐	☐	☐	Hyperactive	Moderate	Dull, slow
Emotions	☐	☐	☐	Anxiety, fear, uncertainty	Anger, hate, jealousy	Calm, greedy, attachment
Faith	☐	☐	☐	Variable	Extremist	Consistent
Intellect	☐	☐	☐	Quick but faulty response	Accurate response	Slow, exact
Recollection	☐	☐	☐	Recent good, remote poor	Distinct	Slow and sustained
Dreams	☐	☐	☐	Quick, active, many, fearful	Fiery, war, violence	Lakes, snow, romantic
Sleep	☐	☐	☐	Scanty, broken up, sleeplessness	Little but sound	Deep, prolonged
Speech	☐	☐	☐	Rapid, unclear	Sharp, penetrating	Slow, monotonous
Financial	☐	☐	☐	Poor, spends on trifles	Spends money on luxuries	Rich, good money preserver
TOTAL						

©1994, 2016 excerpted from *Ayurvedic Cooking for Self-Healing* by Usha and Dr. Lad.
The Ayurvedic Institute • P.O. Box 23445 • Albuquerque, NM 87192-1445 • (505) 291-9698 • www.ayurveda.com

Now before we can look at how to boost your energy and maintain wellness, you first need to establish what 'good health' is. According to Ayurveda, there are certain signs which indicate a person is healthy, they are as follows:

- Can fall asleep and maintain deep sleep.
- Wake up feeling refreshed in the morning.
- Has a good appetite for food and experiences hunger at regular intervals.
- Digests the ingestion of food in its appropriate time, light meals 1-2 hours, heavy meals 3-4 hours.
- Urinates on regular intervals and quantity.
- Opens bowels regularly, at least 1-2 daily.
- Release flatus and burps at regular intervals.
- Has good energy and glowing skin.
- Can hear, see, taste, feel, touch and smell clearly.
- Considers all living beings equal.
- Follows truth, lives in honesty, integrity and with active compassion.
- Has a pleasant mind with controlled emotions.
- Performs charity.
- On waking your tongue is pink. If you have white furry substance on your tongue, then you have ama (toxins) in your body.

A coated tongue (ama) indicates undigested nutrients. This is usually predominant first thing in the morning. Ama is the toxic material that interferes with the free movement of things in the body. It acts as a poison and influences body, organs and systems, primarily slowing down digestion and assimilation of nutrients.

> *Ama is the toxic material that interferes with the free movement of things in the body.*

When ama is present, it is more difficult to make the right decisions and determine right judgments because the mind is not thinking clearly. This can happen at any age.

Removing the ama will remove the disease, and this will recharge and renew damaged tissue over time.

Ama and treatment

Ayurveda considers Ama to be the main cause of all disease. The literal meaning of the word *ama* is undigested. This usually comes about through low digestive fire (Agni), poor food combinations and choices, inadequate elimination of wastes or because the Doshas are out of balance.

Ama is a sticky substance which blocks the natural flow and process within our body. Ama will exacerbate the Doshas which centralise into the stomach for removal via the mouth and anus. Ama (toxins) will weaken Agni (digestive fire), which will in turn, result in producing disease in the weakest parts of the body.

Ama is characterised by having a white fluffy tongue on inspection in the morning before any food or fluids.

Signs of Ama in the body:
- Feeling heavy and lethargic.
- White coated tongue in the morning.
- Disturbed digestion.
- Headaches.
- Concentrated urine.
- Sticky, offensive smelling stools.
- Constipation, swelling and bloating.
- Localised or generalised pain in the body.
- Low physical and mental energy.
- Not fresh on waking in the morning.

- After lunch, person feel heavy and will often take a short nap.
- On rising in the morning, you experience stiffness and heaviness.

How to eliminate Ama

- Tongue scrape first thing in the morning before any food, fluids or brushing your teeth. Ama is predominant first thing in the morning.
- Drink warm water with the juice of half a lemon squeezed into the warm water.
- Administer self-body massage with room temperature oil after shower. Oil massage all orifices. This will stimulate the tissues, promoting movement and digestion of ama.
- Eat at the right time of day in accordance with the season and your Dosha type.
- Heat and exercise helps in the movement of ama.
- Spices stimulate digestive fire (Agni). The stronger your Agni is, the better the elimination of ama.
- For one day per week, have just warm fluids. This is easily digestible and will rest the body.
- Eat a good breakfast, main meal at noon and evening light meal before 7pm.
- Be in bed by 10.30pm to produce healthy sleep cycles for rejuvenation and repair of the body.

The Four Pillars of Health

To be in a state of constant wellness, you need to have a strong constitution and functional support system. Ayurveda refers to this as the Four Pillars of Health. They are nutrition, rest, relationships and exercise. All of these are essential as they interconnect with each other.

Nutrition

Nourishment has always been synonymous with nutrition. Nourishment not only comes from nutritious food, but also clean water and pure air. 'You are what you eat': how many times have you seen this advertised or heard it from others? Countless, I'm sure. Well, this statement is probably the most accurate in terms of correlation with Ayurveda philosophy - fresh is best as it is full of energetic goodness known as prana. Once food is cooked, it starts to deteriorate. After thirty minutes, it loses its nutrients, making it hard to digest. All meals should be eaten as soon as they are cooked for goodness and flavour. The longer food is refrigerated and reheated, the less nutritious it is. Ideally, all food should be consumed at meal times and any food left over should be given to those who are less fortunate.

> *...the mind is involved in food preferences, if you eat what you do not like, then the body will not digest fully.*

"Food gives strength, stamina and stability. This promotes growth, energy, repair, body cell maintenance, protects immunity and prevents immune breakdown. Food creates lustrous skin, clear voice, mental efficiency and ability. This gives satisfaction and happiness for a better life with physical, mental and spiritual fitness." **-Professor Dr P H Kulkarni**

It is important to understand that because the mind is involved in food preferences, if you eat what you do not like then the body will not digest it fully. As a conscience spiritual being, it is your responsibility to choose foods to eat that are useful and beneficial to body-mind.

Protein is needed to build and maintain body tissues. Reliable sources include eggs, cheese, chicken, lean meats, fish and nuts. Intake of protein should be 10-20% of all meals.

All health starts with good digestion.

Tips for better digestion

- Eat for your Dosha type and season.
- Make right food choices based on Dosha, not desire.
- Keep your digestion fire (Agni) strong as it is seat of most disease.
- Eat at the right time with the right amount of food.
- If digestion is low, avoid cold and raw foods.
- Walk after meals for 10-15 minutes as this aids digestion.
- Eat fresh, seasonal locally grown foods, organic if possible.
- If digestion is sluggish, boost digestion with ½ teaspoon grated ginger, ½ teaspoon lemon juice and a pinch of rock salt 15 minutes before meals.
- Fast one day a week with fluids only, warm soups and herbal teas.
- Start your day with warm water, juice of half a lemon and a pinch of ginger to promote digestion.
- Ideally eat small meals 3-4 times daily.
- Eat a large nutritious breakfast with a variety of ingredients.
- Have your biggest meal in the middle of the day.
- Have your light dinner as early as possible.
- Eat when you are hungry.
- Don't eat if you don't know what's in the food.

- Do not have sex, exercise, study or sleep within one hour of eating.
- Eat organic food, avoid white processed foods.
- Eat food cooked with love.
- Eat only after your previous meal has been digested.
- Use digestive herbs and spices in your cooking (if necessary) e.g. ginger, cumin, garlic, cardamom, cinnamon, fennel, fenugreek, rosemary, peppermint, dill, aniseed and caraway.
- Chew all food thoroughly before swallowing.
- Wash your hands before preparing food and dining.
- Eat in a quiet, clean, pleasant environment.
- Never eat while reading or in front of television or computer, sitting down to eat should be a ritual, soft music is good.
- Give thanks of gratitude before meals.
- Eat in good light and ventilation with good company.
- Drink warm water with your meals, sipping occasionally.
- Limit talking while eating as this distracts you from absorbing every flavour.
- Include in each meal, roughly: protein 10-20%, grains 20% and vegetables 60-70%.
- Meat is not recommended to be eaten more than 1-2 times a week and needs to be cooked well in the form of soups and casseroles for easy digestion.
- Do not eat when bored, angry, depressed, emotionally upset, with a disturbed mind, in tension or after exercise.
- Never waste food, any leftover share with others, pets and plants.
- After eating to aid digestion chew 1 tsp of equal amounts of fennel seeds, cumin seeds, cardamom seeds, black pepper and rock salt.

- Massage stomach in an anticlockwise direction with warm oil to aid in digestion.
- Ayurveda suggests filling the stomach ½ with solids, ¼ with water (sips during the meal) and to leave a quarter free.

Recipes for all body types

BREAKFAST

IRON-RICH YOGHURT DRINK
¼ cup raisins
¼ cup unsulfured dried apricots, peaches or figs
1 cup water
½ cup plain low-fat yoghurt

Soak raisins and dried fruit overnight in water. In morning blend all ingredients together mixing well.

SCRAMBLED TOFU
½ package tofu cut into cubes
1 Tbsp ghee
¼ tsp mustard seeds
¼ tsp turmeric
⅛ tsp asafoetida
¼ tsp sea salt
¼ tsp black pepper
⅛ tsp ground cumin

Warm the ghee in a heavy pan. Add mustard seeds and heat till they pop. Add tofu and after lightly frying mash with a fork into small pieces. Add rest of ingredients stirring well. Cook for 3-5 minutes on medium heat.

BREAKFAST BAGEL
½ Whole-wheat bagel toasted
1 egg
1 tsp apple cider
2 slice tomatoes

2 slice avocados
2oz low fat soft cheese

Boil water and apple cider lightly in a pan.
Place avocado and cheese onto toasted bagel.
Poach egg. Crack into boiled water and cook for 5 minutes or until yolk is firm.
Remove egg from boil and place on top of bagel.
Season with salt and pepper and serve.

LUNCH

BAKED RICOTTA
4 Tbsp olive oil
1 tsp paprika
½ tsp sea salt
1 tsp tarragon leaves
½ tsp turmeric
Ground black pepper
Mix all the above together in a bowl
375gm fresh ricotta slice

Place ricotta on an oiled tray and baste with the herb and spice mixture from the bowl. Baste all over including sides. Bake in a moderate oven 180 C for about ¾ hour, basting several times throughout with the remaining mixture. When lightly brown remove and allow to cool before serving with salad.

CUMIN ZUCCHINI MUSHROOMS
2 medium zucchinis
3 shiitake mushrooms
2 Tbsp ghee
½ tsp whole cumin seeds

Soak mushrooms in a cup of water for 10 minutes or until tender. Heat ghee in pan, add cumin seeds, and fry until brown. Wash and slice zucchini. Drain and slice mushrooms. Add zucchini and mushrooms to ghee mixture and stir. Cook for 5 minutes on medium heat.

VEGETABLE SUBJI (DISH)
2 Tbsp ghee
¼ tsp asafoetida
1 Tbsp fresh grated ginger
1 tsp cumin seeds
½ tsp fennel seeds

Recommended vegetables are precooked: cauliflower, potato, and fresh spinach, capsicum, peas, tomato or zucchini.

Heat ghee, add spices and fry gently. When slightly brown and fragrant, add vegetables and toss through the mixture coating them well.

SOUPS

LEEK SOUP
2 Tbsp oil
½ tsp asafoetida powder
3 leeks washed and chopped
1 Tbsp flour
2 dollops cream
1 litre water
2 vegetable stock cubes (dilute in water)
1 Tbsp. lemon juice
½ tsp ground cloves
3-4 drops soy sauce
1 cup sour cream

Salt and pepper to taste

Heat oil in a large heavy pan, add in asafoetida and fry for a couple of seconds. Fry leeks in the pan for a few minutes, add in flour and pour in stock.

Boil for 10 minutes then blend in food processor. Return to boil, whisk in cream then add salt, pepper, cloves, soy sauce and lemon juice. Mix sour cream with some liquid from the pan and whisk into a soup. Serve warm with croutons and dollop of sour cream on top.

KUMARA AND LENTIL SOUP
2 tsp oil
1 small chopped onion
1 medium chopped kumara
½ cup red lentils
1 large vegetable stock cube
3 cups water

Heat the oil in large saucepan on a medium heat. Add in onion and stir till onion is soft. Add in remaining ingredients, bring it to the boil then reduce the heat to simmer for 20 minutes or until kumara is soft. Cover the saucepan. Blend mixture until smooth. Serve warm and garnish with parsley and yoghurt.

CREAM OF CURRIED VEGETABLE AND SPLIT PEA SOUP
4-5 Tbsp ghee or good vegetable oil
1 Tbsp curry powder
½ cup finely chopped onion
½ cup finely chopped carrots
½ cup finely chopped carrots
1 cup water

¾ cup pureed fresh tomatoes (or ½ cup tomato puree)
3 cups cooked split peas or chana dhal
¼ tsp black pepper
Salt to taste
½ - ¾ cup light cream or milk
Chopped coriander to garnish

Heat the ghee or oil in a deep pot on a medium-high heat. When the pot is very hot, add the curry powder, onion, carrots and celery. Sauté the vegetables for 5 minutes till they brown evenly. Add 1 cup water, tomatoes, split peas, pepper and salt.

Cover and cook for 10 minutes until vegetables are tender. Stir in cream or milk to give the soup a smooth velvet consistency. Heat well and garnish with chopped fresh coriander.

DINNER

BEETROOT CURRY
3-4 beetroot sliced into sticks
2 Tbsp dry roasted curry powder
1 Tbsp ground coriander
1 tsp fenugreek powder
1 tsp turmeric
1 tsp salt
½ tsp paprika
10 curry leaves
1 can of coconut milk
Mix all together in a bowl.
3 Tbsp ghee
1 pinch asafoetida
1 tbsp. cumin seeds
I cup water

Heat the ghee, asafoetida and cumin together. Fry for a few minutes till fragrant. Add all the ingredients you mixed in a bowl toss and fry gently for a few minutes. Add water; bring to boil and then simmer for 1 hour (or place in oven covered)

DAHL
1¾ cups whole/split mung bean (soaked overnight, drain in the morning)
6½ cups water
1 Tbsp ghee
½ tsp mustard seeds
½ tsp turmeric
1 tsp sea salt
⅛ Asafoetida
1 ½ tsp barley malt or brown rice syrup
1 ½ tsp lime or lemon juice
1 tsp coriander powder
½ tsp cinnamon
¼ tsp mild curry powder

In a heavy saucepan heat ghee and add mustard seeds. When the mustard seeds pop, add turmeric, asafoetida, mung beans and remaining ingredients. Mix well. Cover and cook for ½ hour if split mung and 1 hour if whole mung beans are used. Test to see if mung beans are soft. If so, ready to serve with chapattis (Indian bread) or basmati rice. Serves 6.

KHICHADI
1 Cup   Basmati rice
½ Cup Split mung beans (split yellow colour)
½ tsp Turmeric
6 Cups Water
Pinch of asafoetida powder

Combine rice and mung beans and wash three times. Add this to boiling water, along with turmeric and asafoetida.
Cook over a medium heat uncovered until all the water is absorbed. Once absorbed, add a further cup of water.
Reduce to a low heat and cook for a further 5 minutes uncovered until all water is absorbed.

You may add additional spices to taste at this point cooking for a further few minutes to allow the spices to be infused into the rice.

Consistency should be like stew and very moist.

Recommended spices for Khichadi: Basil, black pepper, coriander, cumin, dill and fennel.

DESSERTS

SPICED PEARS
5 ripe medium pears (about 4 cups chopped)
½ cup apricot nectar
¼ cup water
1/8 tsp dry ginger
3 cloves
1 pod cardamom or 3 cardamom seeds
Pinch sea salt

Wash, quarter and core pears. Chop in pieces. Put all ingredients in saucepan and cook uncovered over medium heat for 15 minutes or until soft. Serve hot. Serves 4.

TAPIOCA HALVA
1 Cup tapioca
1½ cups of coconut milk (soak both these ingredients overnight)

Boil 1 cup sugar in ½ cup water and ½ cup unsalted butter and 10-15 saffron threads. Add tapioca mix and cook, stirring constantly till mixture leaves the side of the pan. Spread in tray and press roasted cashews on top.

VANILLA CUSTARD
250ml soy milk
1 Tbsp cornflour
1 tsp vanilla essence

Combine all ingredients in a small saucepan over a medium heat. Whisk until thickened then pour into 2 small bowls and cool before serving.

Serve with shortbread, carrot, banana or other fruit.

BEVERAGES

MANGO COCONUT SMOOTHIE
Flesh from 1 large mango
1 ¾ cups coconut milk
1 ½ Tbsp fresh lime juice
2 Tbsp sugar

Add all ingredients in a blender and mix for 1-2 minutes. Drink immediately. May serve this chilled.

ROSE LASSI
1 cup vanilla yoghurt
2 cups water
1 tsp rose water

Blend together, serve slightly chilled, garnish with organic rose petals.

CHAI
Cloves
Cardamom pods
Cinnamon sticks
Lemongrass
Ginger fresh is best
Black Tea or rooibos tea
Milk
Palm sugar or jaggary to taste
Boil water with black tea
Grind spices and add to tea
Add the milk and palm sugar or jaggary to taste.

RASAYANA (TONIC) DRINK
To be taken at night before bed if elderly or recovering from illness.

5-10 saffron threads (soak for 5-10mins)
2 Tb hot water
1 cup milk (un-homogenised) (use any other alternative milk except soy. If you are lactose intolerant don't use cow's milk.)
1-2 tsp ghee
½-1 tsp organic honey

Soak saffron in hot water, then add to milk and bring to the boil.

When milk froths, wait 30sec until froth subsides and boil again. Repeat again so it is boiled 3 times.
Remove from heat and allow for cooling, (this is done by pouring cup to cup).
When less than lukewarm (i.e. 40 deg) add honey.

Stir in a clock wise direction. Drink quickly. Don't sip.
Add cinnamon or nutmeg to taste.
Sit quietly for 5-10mins after drinking.

NEVER add equal amounts of honey and ghee therefore:
½ tsp honey to 1tsp ghee
1tsp honey to 2 tsp ghee
1 tsp honey to ½ tsp ghee

Equal amounts are ama increasing, i.e. toxic.

Rest

Sleep is fundamental to life. It is essential for the proper functioning of the body and the mind. Without adequate restful sleep, the body will experience sleep deprivation. This will result in a decreased ability to concentrate, perform complex tasks, communicate and listen effectively.

Sufficient sleep is 5-10 hours a night, depending on individual needs. Most people will sleep an average of eight hours. Children usually need 10-12 hours for growth, whereas the elderly usually survive happily on 5-6 hours a night.

> *Sleep is essential for the proper functioning of the body and the mind.*

Anyone who is unwell or recovering from illness requires more sleep, as this allows for the body to grow, repair, recuperate and revitalise.

Activities to be applied to help maintain adequate sleep:

- Your evening meal should be light and/or of a fluid consistency and eaten by 7pm.
- Go for a light walk after meals.
- Stop eating at least two hours before retiring.
- May have warmed milk with cinnamon or nutmeg to taste.
- Warm oil massage to head and feet after warm bath.
- Make sure your bed is comfortable with adequate linen.
- Your bedroom has soothing colours (pastels of greens, blues, lilacs and beige (no red please as this disturbs sleep).
- Your sleeping environment is well ventilated and comfortably warm.
- Soft music and slight fragrance may be used.

- Avoid the use of television and computer devices in your bedroom.
- Best time to retire is between 9-10pm. By 11pm the body will get a second wind and you feel like you're in 1999 party mode. It is important to be well rested and asleep by then, so if this is not your habit, then you need to retrain your brain.
- The body does its repair work between 2-4am so it is important you are not awake at this time.
- The head of your bed should be facing east or south to optimise sleep.
- Signs of a good sleep is feeling refreshed on waking.

Relationships

- Relationships are the cornerstone of human existence. Without them we cannot grow into ourselves.
- Studies have been done on premature babies in incubators that do not have physical contact with another human being; the baby develops a condition called 'failure to thrive'. Failure to thrive is when a baby loses or cannot gain their expected weight. This also happens a lot in babies that have been neglected or abused. This is a result of the loss of emotional bond between parent and child.
- Once the baby is held and stroked on a regular basis then they start to gain weight. Healthy human connection with others is vital for good health.

The first relationship we need to have to become vibrant and healthy as adults, is the relationship with ourselves. This entails knowing and understanding all aspects of ourselves, so

> ...the first relationship we need to have to become vibrant and healthy as adults, is the relationship with ourselves...

we can shine and be a star in our life. Once we understand what drives us, our strengths, how we are challenged, and what our pleasures and needs are, only then can we attract a partner where we can maintain an intimate and loving relationship.

The second relationships we need to be healthy, are adult to adult relationships. They require self-understanding, patience, commitment, shared core values, honest communication, respect, discernment, chemistry, caring, love and a solid foundation in integrity.

Any relationship that suffers with poor boundaries, lack of integrity, poor communication, abuse, lack of love and affection will contribute to stress which will lead to dysfunction and ultimately disease.

If this is the case, then individual and or couple's therapy is recommended to re-establish the original relations.

The third relationship you have is the one with the environment. As change is the only constant in life, as part of health management you need to be at one with your surroundings. When the external environment changes, your internal environment needs to adapt accordingly. If this transition takes place easily then you have an innate good stress response in which you learn something of value. If you are unwilling to adapt you cause a bad stress response that contributes to weakening your immune system and will eventually lead to *dis-ease*.

Exercise

Exercise is defined as an act or movement that causes breathing to become deeper and the body to start to perspire. Regular exercise will maintain weight and keep the whole body's circuitry functioning at peak levels. It also increases mental acuity, improves complexion, regulates metabolism and digestive power and aids in the growth of muscles and limbs. A strong body will also give your body the ability to endure fatigue.

Recommended exercises include walking, short jogs, dancing, yoga, tennis, football, basketball and swimming. Exercise should not be in excess as this can increase weakness in the body if you are not in good condition. It is the widespread belief that you go to the gym to get healthy. This is *not* true. Without good health and a well-functioning body, you only put your body under further stress causing further dis-ease. As an example, if you suffer with chronic fatigue or depression, as much as we all know exercise will increase energy, your body just does not have the physical capacity to partake in exercise until your body heals. Your body and mindset need to be healthy before you undertake any sports or gym work. Consult your medical practitioner before commencing excessive exercise.

> *Your body and mindset need to be healthy before you undertake any sports of gym work.*

Exercise is contraindicated in the following circumstances:

- Immediately after a meal.
- Immediately after sex.
- When you are thirsty.
- Those who are emotionally upset.
- Acute inflammatory conditions such as infection, fever or stress.

A personalised program is recommended for the following:

- Persons afflicted with disease or pain.
- Weak persons.
- Those suffering from chronic disease.

Tips for optimum exercise:

- Exercise is best performed before meals or 2-3 hours after eating.
- Exercise to your Dosha (Vata, Pitta or Kapha) type and energy level, increasing as desired and able.
- Over-exercise depletes the body's available energy and can cause permanent damage.
- Perform high intensity exercises in winter and low intensity in summer.

Being a productive individual in society promotes a sense of identity and self-esteem. Your occupation is exercise for your brain and your body (depending on your occupation type). Most people work 8-10 hours a day (including travelling time). Approximately 40% of your daily time is dedicated to this activity. With this amount of time and energy devoted to your profession, being happy with your work goes a long way to being healthy in your body.

If you hold a position which deals with stress as part of the package, then it is your responsibility to ask for the tools and techniques you need to manage the stress productivity. This may come in the form of stress management classes; having power naps; using an open communication style; including massage or exercise at lunchtime and organising and prioritising your day;

Your chosen occupation should be satisfying, allowing for personal growth.

learning deep breathing: the inhale breath energises the body and the exhale breath relaxes the body.

Your chosen occupation should be satisfying, allowing for personal growth. Feelings of satisfaction and fulfilment help promote a healthy immune system keeping you free from disease. *Live what you love.*

Daily Routine (Dinacharya)

Maintaining your health is a matter of practising good habits daily. This is more effective than periodic detoxification or fasting.

Getting into a regular ritual will bring many benefits in your life and will optimise your wellbeing. Once there is a strong daily routine in place, then this becomes your path of least resistance because it becomes habit forming and regular.

It is advantageous to start any new routine at the new moon or full moon as this is the point of creation of new energy.

Morning

- A healthy adult should rise 60-90 minutes before sunrise. This is the time to practice meditation, yoga and deep breathing.
- Practice of ritual or worship and/or religious prayer.
- Drink warm water and lemon juice to aid digestion.
- Bowels and bladder should be completely emptied.
- Stools should be easily evacuated and should sink. If they float this is an indication that your digestion is low/weak, and you have undigested food in your stool known as ama. You may also have gas or fats in your stool.

- Face and eyes should be washed in cool medicated water.
- Scrape the tongue to remove the furry white surface known as ama which is poison to your body if swallowed. This helps to remove waste products and bad odour in the mouth. Use a silver or copper tongue scraper found in most Indian grocers or from an Ayurvedic practitioner.
- Clean the teeth in the morning and after every meal.
- Gargle the mouth with warm water.
- Address all shaving needs.
- Conduct self-massage to body with warm oil, sesame is best. Start at top of the head and work towards the feet. Massage delays aging, improves muscle tone, detoxifies the body and relieves fatigue.
- Take warm cleansing shower or bath.
- Exercise your voice (in the shower is suitable).
- Apply medicated oil (Anu Taila) to nose and ears.
- Dress appropriately for the weather and season.
- Drink warm water with lemon and pinch of ginger for digestion before meals.
- Eat a nutritious breakfast based on your constitution and season.
- Breakfast should have protein and fibre content. Plain yoghurt is best taken in the morning.
- Leave for work at a suitable time avoiding traffic or give yourself ample time to reach your destination without experiencing stress.

Afternoon (12.00-3.00pm)

- The largest meal should be eaten now.
- Digestive bitters taken after meals.
- 100 steps should be taken after meals to aid digestion.
- Light nap (no more than 60 minutes) after lunch.

Mid afternoon

Energy is channelled into work or your job now.

Bio rhythms drop between 3-4pm, causing low blood sugar levels. You are prone to eating sweet foods or caffeine to give you that extra 'hit' to get you through the rest of the day. To prevent this, have a portion of protein or soup at 2.45pm. Keep a packet of nuts or raisins in a drawer in the office or in your bag for access.

Evening

- Evening meal should be eaten before 7.30pm.
- Heavy food, dairy and beef should be avoided as digestion slows down now.
- Digestive bitters taken after meals.
- A stroll outdoors is recommended after the meal.
- Activities like dancing, outdoor games and boating are suitable as this will freshen the mind.
- Discuss the day's events with your partner.
- Avoid sex immediately after food.
- Bath or shower and attend to hygiene needs.
- Meditate before sleep 20-30 minutes.
- Rasayana drink can be taken now as this promotes health and wellbeing.
- To secure good night's sleep, retire no later than 10.30pm.

Seasonal Support (Ritucharya)

As much as daily routines are an important part of your health maintenance plan, so is the practice of seasonal routines. As human beings, we interact continuously with our external environment. Because of this we need to adapt as our environment changes from season to season.

Disease states usually occur at junctions of these seasons, so it is advisable to keep in the best of health in all seasons and adapt as needed. They are divided into three seasons; spring, summer and late autumn through to winter.

Spring - Vata season

Spring is known as the allergy season and the birth of all things new. In spring, body resistance and digestion are both compromised.

The parts of the body primarily affected are the stomach, sinuses and lungs. Coughs, colds, congestion and spring allergies are the ailments that come out to play now.

A diet low in fats and oils, lighter and less oily in nature is advisable now. Warm cooked foods are preferable for digestion. Bitter and astringent foods should be added. Dairy products that are mucus forming and heavy foods like banana, avocado, meat and cold drinks, should be avoided.

> *Warm spices like ginger, garlic, cinnamon and black pepper will help break down excessive phlegm and water in the body.*

Drinking warm water with a pinch of ginger and cinnamon in the morning and chewing roasted cumin and fennel seeds after meals will aid digestion.

Warm spices like ginger, garlic, cinnamon and black pepper will help break down excessive phlegm and water in the body.

Detoxification, exercise, gardening, walks in the parks, and oil massage are beneficial now. Wearing cotton in colours of pink, orange, yellow and violet are soothing and suitable for spring.

Avoid sleeping in the daytime, air conditioning, and heavy, cold, oily and sweet foods.

Summer - Pitta season

Summer is the time of heat, surf, sun and tans. In summer, body resistance is minimal, and digestion is weak. The parts of the body primarily affected are the liver and stomach.

Excessive sweating and dehydration may result from the heat. Emotions tend to be volatile now and anger, passion and violent behaviour may be exhibited now. This needs to be channelled productively, so exercise or sports is best early in the morning before the day gets hot. The exception here is swimming, this is better in the evening. Swimming is highly recommended as it cools the body and may be done any time of day. If swimming in salt water, make sure to wash off the salt to prevent a build-up of heat in the body. Make sure you are well-hydrated while exercising.

Overindulgence in the sun can cause overheating. Sunburn and melanoma is one of the leading causes of skin cancer in Australia and New Zealand. As the sun is the enemy now, full protection of hat and sun block should be used. Sunglasses should be used only in the brightest part of the day, as constant wearing of sunglasses decreases your eyesight.

> *Sunglasses should be used only in the brightest part of the day as constant wear of sunglasses decreases your eyesight.*

A hydrating cooling diet like salads and fresh green vegetables are recommended now. Coriander leaf is an excellent cooling herb to add to salads, drinks and yoghurt. Sweet and bitter foods digest well now.

120

Sour, salty and hot foods, hot and spicy spices, alcoholic beverages, caffeine and nicotine all dehydrate the body and should be eliminated or at least limited.

Frequenting cool places, nature and water soothes the soul and cools the mind. Light, loose clothing, cottons and silks in cooling colours of white, grey, blue, purple and green work well in summer.

Walking and sleeping in moonlight gives coolness to the body, sweet cool light liquids, cooled water (not refrigerated), milk, ghee, coconut water, coconut oil body massage and retiring before 10.30pm are all recommended here to keep the body in balance for summer.

Avoid exercise in strong sunlight and excess of sex as heat in the body can be aggravated.

Late Autumn to Winter - Kapha season

In autumn, the leaves change into beautiful golden colours and the winds feel fresh and cool against your face. The weather is changeable with warm days and cool nights.

Body resistance and digestion are both moderate now. In winter, body resistance is at its maximum and digestion is strong.

In this season, the nervous system, the colon, skin and bones are primarily affected.

Foods that are favoured are sweet, sour, salty and oily in taste. Food should be warm, well cooked and easily digested.

> *In this season the nervous system, the colon, skin and bones are primarily affected.*

Soups and casseroles are suitable in this season. Raw vegetables, dry foods, frozen foods and dairy should be avoided along with coriander, fenugreek, parsley and turmeric.

Beverages should be warm, and teas made with warming herbs like cinnamon, clove, ginger and liquorice. Ice drinks, alcohol and ice should be avoided.

Daily meditation and warm oil massage with sesame oil before bedtime helps to promote restful sleep. Camomile tea or warm milk with nutmeg, cinnamon or cardamom is also useful.

Cold winds and draughts, cycling, excessive exercise, driving and flying should all be limited. Exercise should be done indoors.

You should be warm in this season, especially in the chest, so natural fibres such as wool should be used.

Colours of red, orange and yellow should be worn to promote warmth.

How to boost energy by optimising your physiology

- A healthy person needs to have good connections with others and a clear direction on where they are going and how to get there.
- If you live a healthy lifestyle and still feel tired, your digestion may not be assimilating your food thoroughly. You may need to consult your medical/herbal practitioner to determine that you have no parasites in your digestive system. This is often the cause of digestive problems in the majority of cases. Parasites are easily absorbed and may occur more frequently in

people who have pets; those who walk barefoot; live in the country or travel abroad. Parasites in the gut will drain blood from the bowel lining and feed off the nutrients in the food, leaving your body feeling depleted. Parasite cleanse should be done annually to keep digestion tract in good condition.
- Know what foods invigorate you and which foods deplete your energy.
- Make sure your iron levels are sufficient for your daily needs, especially if you are vegetarian, do excessive exercise or are of menstrual age. Reliable sources of iron other than lean meat include green leafy vegetables, sardines and hazelnuts.
- Check your folic acid and vitamin B12 levels whenever you have your annual blood check-up, as this can also cause anaemia.
- Check your thyroid levels as this can also make you feel tired.
- Be sure you are getting 8 hours of restful sleep at night so that you wake up refreshed and energised.
- A brisk walk in sunlight can recharge your batteries as the sun is how the planet is revitalised and people are no different.
- Work your body rhythms with the cycles of a nature.
- Fasting or detoxification at the new and full moons enhances this process.
- Avoid sleeping during the day, especially after a big meal.
- Wearing colours of red, orange and yellow can be energising.
- Aromas of lemon, orange, peppermint and basil are uplifting.
- Breathe in fresh air; allow prana (chi) to circulate throughout your body.

- Eat slow release carbohydrates like beans, wholegrain bread and starchy vegetables as this will sustain your energy levels.
- Avoid quick release carbohydrates like sugar, fizzy drinks and chocolate. This will give an instant surge of energy then drop energy levels sharply, resulting in lethargy and mood swings.
- Regular exercise outside improves oxygenation to the body, stimulates your senses and invigorates you.
- When body-mind becomes disturbed or weakened, disease intervenes, so it is important to deal with any psycho/emotional issues cleanly and efficiently, with clarity; manage your life well and have good thoughts.

The human body thrives when it is loved and taken care of. Practising daily and seasonal good habits will establish the vitality needed to live happily with life's challenges, making right choices that serve you along the way.

> *The human body thrives when it is loved and taken care of.*

People tend to take loving care of their vehicles because they want to be able to reach their destinations safely. So, as part of the car's regular routine, you attend to the right fuel (food as fire) for the vehicle, polish and wash the car (body is earth), maintain annual mechanic check-ups (medical check-ups), check tyre pressure (air), make sure oil and water levels are full (water) and tend to all repairs promptly (illness). This is all part of the car's health for you to feel safe in the vehicle; likewise, the same applies for the human body.

So, in conclusion, what is Ayurveda?

Geographically, Indian medicine.

Historically, the oldest medicine.

Ecologically, the most sustainable medicine.

Philosophically, holistic medicine.

Scientifically, the one medicine that has information that is constantly being proven.

Effectively, the art of blissful living and science of complete healing.

Therapeutically, the purest, fastest, safest and person-centred medicine.

Dr. Rama Prasad BAMS, CACH, Clinical Director at Sydney Ayurveda Centre
SydneyAyurvedaCentre.com

Personal Notes

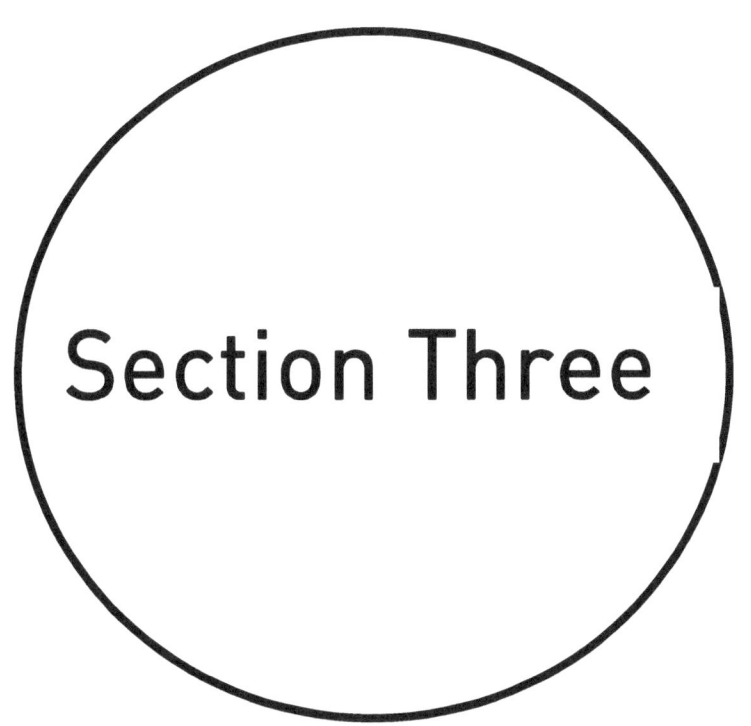

Section Three

Spiritual Health

"When life or energy flows unimpeded and through right direction to its precipitation (the related gland), then the form responds, and ill health disappears" Esoteric Healing, Law VII, Alice A. Bailey.

Energetic Healing

Energetic Healing is also known as Reiki, Healing Touch, Therapeutic Touch, Pranic Healing, Chi, Ki, Bio-energy, Subtle Energy, Spiritual Healing and Hands on Healing. Although the techniques may vary, the basic principles of Energy and Healing are very similar.

Every person has their own unique life force and is unable to exist without one. Similarly, every culture has its own name for that life-force.

- In India, it is known as Prana.
- South Americans call it Gana.
- Japan refers to the force as Ki.
- The Polynesian Islands describe it as Mana.
- In China, the word Qi (Chi) is used.
- Hawaiians identify it as Tane.
- In Western Culture, the terms Subtle energy, Life force and Bio-energy are universally used.

Every culture recognises the powerful energy within each human being, and every culture has its own energetic and healing modalities that provide alignment, balance and wholeness.

Our energy field (or aura) consists of seven layers. It is within the first four layers that most imbalances occur in a person's life. Consequently, this is where energy-based work is usually done. These layers consist of:

Layer one: Etheric or Vital layer (the layer closest to the body).
Layer two: Emotional layer.
Layer three: Mental layer.
Layer four: Intuitive, astral or spiritual layer.
Layer five: Etheric template.
Layer six: Celestial body.
Layer seven: Ketheric body.

Once the practitioner is grounded, and have set their intention, they then extend their energy and connect to the Universal Energy Field. This energy then resonates through the healer and back to the client's energy field. This technique is non-invasive and creates significant changes in the physical, emotional, mental and spiritual dimensions.

Energy healing

- induces relaxation, thus promoting self-healing. It accelerates the healing process of wounds resulting from surgery or trauma.

- Reduces stress, anxiety and assists pain relief.

- Clears the mind and aids in the recovery of depression.

- Keeps the body-mind integrated and grounded.

- Aids in restoration and maintenance of energy levels and enhances spiritual growth.

- Is beneficial in preparing the body for surgery, therefore minimising post-operative effects.

- Maintains a healthy immune system.

- Supports the process of grief and dying.

Dis-ease of the body is an indication that a person's energy system is blocked or out of alignment. Dis-ease starts in the energetic body first, which consists of a network of chakras within our energy field (or aura). Signs and symptoms present themselves in the physical body because of this.

The word Chakra comes from the Sanskrit meaning 'wheel' and this wheel is noted on the Indian flag as the country's mark of spirituality. "The chakras are in the nature of disturbing agencies and electric batteries, providing dynamic force and qualitative energy to man." *Djwhal Khul, as channelled through Alice A. Bailey.*

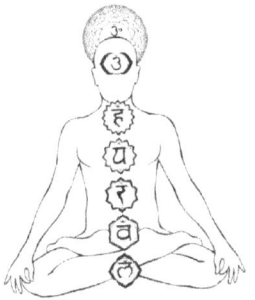

Chakra positions

Chakras are wheels of light that spin in your auric field creating their own electromagnetic field which can be measured. They work as a system, in harmony and in connection with each other, spinning at their own vibration. To maintain optimum health, all chakras must be spinning in the same direction and at the same speed, aligned with each other.

Any blocks: physical, emotional, physiological and/or spiritual will cause disturbance and throw the chakra system out of vibration and sequence. The chakras are connected via the nadis system. Chakras correlate directly to the endocrine glands in our physical body and the connection is via the nervous system. If a chakra is over or under stimulated, the chakra spins in excess and the person can manifest signs and symptoms of the chakra indicating imbalance.

Some people have a dominant chakra. The chakra dominates their daily lives and therefore, it becomes over stimulated. For example: if a person is constantly angry and exhibits violent behaviour, then their third chakra that sits in the solar plexus, their seat of personal power, is overstimulated. Likewise, the same in reverse, if the chakra is under stimulated or recessive, the person may exhibit signs of low self-esteem and lack of courage. They will be unable to assert their personal power and will experience feelings of unworthiness. While in this energetic state, they will attract persons or situations into their life that will reinforce their belief of unworthiness until they find it in their own personal power.

When one chakra is affected, it is normal for the chakra above it and the one below it to also be unbalanced. Chakras work in sequence and alignment with each other, affecting the whole body. When they are in harmony and resonating at similar vibrations, the result will be a disease-free body.

There are seven major chakras which are aligned up and down the spine. However, in some Asian cultures, eleven major chakras are identified. Refer to *Miracles through Pranic Healing* by Master Choa Kok Sui for additional information.

Each chakra has a direct correlation to an endocrine gland. When imbalances occur within that chakra, the relevant endocrine gland will also be affected, and can manifest in disease in that area of the body and its surrounding organs.

For this book, I will only focus on the seven major chakras that are situated from the base of the spinal cord to the top of the head.
- Chakras one to three are known as the physical chakras that support your right to exist, create and to manifest the fruits of your labour.
- Chakras five to seven are the spiritual chakras that correlate to your expression of truth, intuition and your connection with your higher self.
- The heart, chakra four, unites and connects the system with compassion, forgiveness, joy and love for yourself and others. Hence when you experience loss or grief, the rest of your body can become unwell.

Chakra One

Responsibility, respond to your ability – Christina Richter

Muladhara - commonly known as the root chakra - is located at the base of spine, connected to the adrenals and rules support and survival. This is the chakra responsible for creating the foundation for life, survival, security, providing for physical needs, grounding, health and standing up for oneself as well as connection to family or tribe.

Signs of imbalance include constipation, obesity, leg and knee problems, osteoarthritis, incapable of being still, financial difficulty, fatigue and fear of life. Can be addicted to food, gambling, shopping and work.

Recommended Healing for Muladhara

Energy flows up through the soles of the feet, up the legs, into the base chakra and up the spinal column, energising all the chakras along the way. This keeps the body in balance and well grounded.

The following are suggestions to keep the base chakra opened, energy flowing through you, with solid foundation:

- Stand (with no shoes on) on grass, earth or sand for ten minutes, twice a day.
- Wear red undergarments and socks. The base chakra is energised by red.
- Eat regularly: red foods and fluids e.g. beetroot, tomato, red apples, red berries, cherries, plums, watermelon, red kidney beans, red lentils radishes, red wine. Have foods with a high concentration of iron e.g. red meat and green leafy vegetables. Eat cooked root vegetables e.g. potatoes, carrot, turnips, and pumpkin.

- Exercise: daily walking, gym work, jogging, martial arts, yoga or dance.
- Regular warm oil massage keeps you in your body.
- Wear the colours of nature; green browns, for balance and integration of your body, no blue.
- Work with your hands in a practical manner e.g. gardening, cooking, massage, woodwork or pottery, playing with young children.
- Understand your fear and move through it.

Develop a routine that works for you, using two or three of these as a daily practice. This will energise you, so you may experience increased vigour, a better self-esteem and increased confidence. Be mindful, if overstimulated, reduce the practices.

Chakra Two

Do what you love and flourish from it. - Christina Richter

Svadhisthana - located between the pubis and navel, is connected to the ovaries and testes and rules sexual creativity. The second chakra is in the sacral area and is primarily concerned with expansion, creative expression and pleasure, emotional and sexual balance within relationships.

Signs of imbalance lower back pain, reproductive complaints, bladder, kidney troubles, unbalanced sex drive, guilt, feelings of isolation and emotional instability. Can be addicted to alcohol, sex and heroin.

Recommended Healing for Svadhisthana
- Reconnect to your inner child and learn to play.
- Allow pleasure to be an abundant part of life.
- Ask for your sexual needs to be met.
- Maintain healthy boundaries.
- Include regular movement like dance and yoga.
- Nourish yourself through your creativity.
- Resolve any guilt issues you may have.

Chakra Three

Accept who you are and be the best you can be – Christina Richter

Manipura - located above the navel, is connected to the pancreas gland, and rules personal will, personal power and self-esteem. The third chakra is located at the solar plexus and relates to ego, personal power, autonomy, physical energy, metabolism, drive, courage and personal will. This provides a keen sense of self-esteem and self-respect when healthy.

Signs of imbalance include ulcers, allergies, digestive disorders, liver and gallbladder ailments, low vitality, misplaced anger, control issues, sensitivity to criticism, low self-esteem, introversion and shame. Can be addicted to amphetamines, cocaine, caffeine, work and anger.

Recommended Healing for Manipura
- Accept yourself and your body.
- Be the best you can be and be proud in it.
- Exercise rigorously if you have a problem containing anger and avoid the colour red.
- Be strong in your own personal power.
- Empower others.
- Establish confidence and assertion.
- Laugh more.

Chakra Four

Love is sharing the self without losing yourself – Christina Richter

Anahata - located in the chest, is connected to the thymus gland and rules compassion, love, and relationships. The fourth chakra is about the heart; the joy, love and relationship a person has with thy self. It also encompasses an individual's sense of personal values, self-acceptance and self-compassion. Only when this is achieved, can you extend real love to others.

Signs of imbalance: all heart related diseases, high blood pressure, mistrust, holding onto past hurts, melancholic, grief and unable to give and receive freely. Can be addicted to tobacco, sugar, love and marijuana.

Recommended Healing for Anahata
- Accept and love yourself.
- Forgive those that have hurt you.
- Let go of past pains as they no longer serve you.
- Allow others to love you and let love in.
- Establish intimacy with people close to you.
- Avoid co-dependant relationships.
- Work through any grief or loss with a counsellor.

Chakra Five

To express yourself and to be heard is your right, from birth
– Christina Richter

Vishuddha - located in the throat and is connected to the thyroid and parathyroid gland, and rules creative self-expression. The fifth chakra governs our communication. It also covers speaking the truth, and a person's sense of choice and freewill.

Signs of imbalance include speech impediments, sore throat, cough, neck problems, laryngitis, thyroid imbalance, respiratory and/or hearing problems and an inability or reluctance to honour the truth. Can be addicted to opiates and Marijuana.

Recommended Healing for Vishuddha
- Practice Pranayama (breath work) daily.
- Start a journal and write daily.
- Play a wind instrument.
- Ask for concrete facts when making decisions.
- Sing in the shower and in the car.
- Speak your truth without fear.
- Wear blue around your throat when speaking in a group.

Chakra Six

People change when they have new insights or perceptions
- Christina Richter

Ajna - located between the eyebrows, connected to the pituitary gland and is the chakra that rules intuition and wisdom. Known as the brow, the sixth chakra's role is to link the sense of knowing or intuition, with wisdom, emotional intelligence, psychic awareness, dreams and visions. Developing the ability to trust this chakra will allow you to see the big picture with heightened intuition and enhanced optimism.

Signs of imbalance include headaches, problems with the Central Nervous System, optical imbalance and hallucination. Can be addicted to hallucinogens and marijuana.

Recommended Healing for Ajna
- Trust your intuition.
- Learn to discern illusion from fact.
- Connect to your intuition through meditation.
- Express yourself through visual creativity.
- Spend time near or in water. Alternatively bring a water feature into your home.
- Heal any trauma with past life regression.
- Be open and trust what you perceive and receive.

Chakra Seven

Wisdom is the ability to see beyond reality – Christina Richter

Sahasrara - located at the top of the head, connected to the pineal gland and rules liberation. The seventh chakra is the one that connects to the higher self or universal truth. It includes an expanded consciousness and the individual's sense of spiritual wisdom. This is the integration point of a person's sense of being and where it aligns with their soul. It is essentially, the core of a person's being.

Signs of imbalance include confusion, depression, obsessive behaviour, an inability to learn, issues with attachment, epilepsy and dementia. Can be addicted to religion and spiritual practices.

Recommended Healing Sahasrara
- Allow more flow into your life.
- Trust in the divine design.
- Release what have no control over.
- Allow yourself to be in stillness.
- Ask for universal guidance and support.
- Declutter your life of belongings and people that you no longer need.
- Develop a spiritual philosophy and/or practice that works for you.

We are spiritual beings in physical bodies. We need to honour both human laws and spiritual laws with love in order in exist in harmony with others, our environment and within ourselves.

Colour meditation

This exercise is designed to balance all your chakras. When done daily (best after your shower), you will feel grounded, protected, have increased vitality and clarity.

- Sit comfortably in loose clothes with feet firmly on the ground and with a straight back.
- Have soft peaceful music in the background and gently close your eyes.
- Clear your mind and take three breathes in through your nose normally. With each breath, you relax more into yourself.
- Concentrate on the soles of your feet.
- Visualise red energy coming through the ground to the soles of your feet and into your ankles.
- Feel the warming sensation of Red -Tomato Red.
- Visualise the Red flowing up to the knees, then thighs and into the base sexual chakra.
- Take a breath through your nose and visualise the colour of an Orange - bring this colour down to an area above the sexual centre and below your umbilicus area (2nd chakra).
- Breathe out from your stomach, through your nose, the colour grey. Do this, three times.
- Breathe in through your nose - warm yellow, sun energy, to the solar plexus area. Breathe out grey energy. Do this, three times.
- Breathe in through your nose, grass green energy. Circulate this energy around your heart. Breathe out grey energy through your nose. Do this, three times.
- Breathe in sky blue energy to your throat area.
- Breathe out grey energy. Do this, three times.
- Breathe in violet purple energy to the point between your eyebrows, your third eye. Breathe out grey energy. Do this, three times.
- Visualise a jug of gold white energy above you.
- Pour the contents of this jug over you.
- Allow your body, organs, cells and aura to totally immerse in the colour of gold and white.
- Take normal breathes, slowly.
- Open eyes when ready and say the following in a mirror three times:
- "I am complete, I am abundant, I am love."
- Follow this with a tall glass of water and commence your day.

Personal Notes

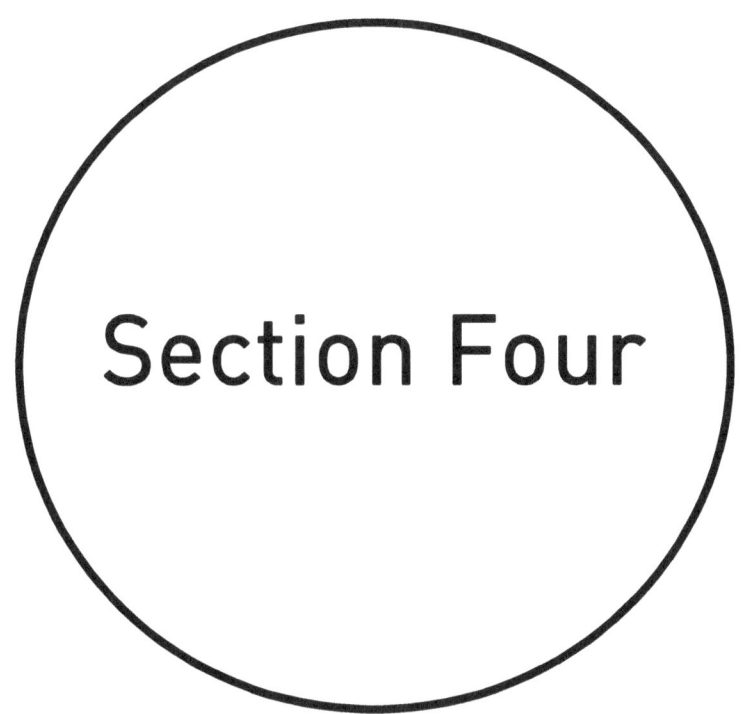

Section Four

Modalities of Healing

"Give yourself permission to nurture yourself; your soul will love you and your body will heal you." – Christina Richter

The ability to self-heal comes from your awareness to self-care. As we are energetic/spiritual beings in physical bodies, there is a need to honour, nurture and integrate both aspects of ourselves equally to achieve and maintain wholeness and wellness.

Your soul works in synergy with your physical body to help achieve your life purpose. When your soul is not nurtured, or the soul's needs are not fulfilled, it can manifest as stress and/or loss of direction. If this is not attended to, it can lead to physical breakdown. The body speaks what the soul seeks. Integration - and connection of body-soul is necessary for a balanced life.

Self-care is important in your daily/weekly routine. This enables the body-soul to feel nourished, aligned and grounded. In this healthy state, you can deal with life's stress and drama in a clear and productive manner with minimal effort.

There are many modalities on offer to help you achieve this. Just walk through your local mall or pick up a health magazine and you are bombarded with adverts on massage (and other therapies) and how it makes you feel good etc. That's all well and good, but to understand why it is good for you and how it works in your body to give this effect, is what this section is all about. Once you are armed with this information then you can decide what you and your body-soul needs, as it differs from person to person. Managing your own health enables you to create your own health maintenance plan that works for you.

The following is an episode of a young woman's life and how her living situation led her to a place of awakening and self-discovery.

Anne's Story

I know now that I should have spent time looking after myself first. I thought, "If he is happy, I will be happy", except ill people are rarely happy.

One thought, two thoughts, three. Worried, never ending thoughts. Questioning, *What if that happens again? What would I do?* Gosh, I never want that to happen.

Welcome to the rollercoaster, as adrenalin hits. Shallow breathing, hands twitching, there is a tightness, almost burning feeling across my chest.

Rational thought gone, I am overwhelmed – scared; if it has once, it can happen again. Tears flood my eyes and trickle down my face. My hand now beats my forehead, as I beg the churning thoughts and feelings of fear to stop.

I must be horrible; this wouldn't happen if I wasn't horrible. I must be terrible. I am terrible. I am panicking! On the worst occasion, alone and sleep deprived, I thought dying would be the better option than to continue enduring this endless treadmill. I pleaded with God, "Just take me, please, stop my heart." God didn't.

However, a doctor recognised my problem, and for short term use prescribed Valium. Dosed up, I finally relaxed, I got some sleep. It wasn't my first, and it wouldn't be my last attack.

Everything changed while taking a simple bike ride with my husband on a summer's day in January 2006, four years earlier. There is a twenty-three-year age difference between us, at the time he was 54 and I was 29 years old. Climbing a steep hill, my husband became extremely breathless. He got off his bike. Exhausted, he collapsed on the grass verge next to the footpath. Moments later he was unconscious. I immediately called out for help, which resulted in a woman from a house across the road calling an ambulance.

My husband had now stopped breathing. He made a momentary rasping, gurgling sound as any remaining air left his lungs and his body went stiff. Another woman came to my assistance. "You are not going to die!" I yelled at him, hoping he would hear me.

This woman told me she knew how to do CPR. He started to turn purple. His eyes were blood shot. We could not find a heartbeat. Together, we started to perform CPR. She did the compressions on his heart and I gave mouth to mouth.

I worked, really worked, like I have never worked before. I leaned forward breathing into his mouth, then turning my head to see his chest filled with air and her hands repeatedly pushing down over his heart and sternum. I counted 1000, 2000... We practised this procedure, high on adrenalin for what felt like forever. It was probably about five minutes - to be honest I don't really know. At one point, for a matter of seconds, I became overwhelmed by dizziness, everything was moving left and right. The woman yelled at me, "Don't stop!" Bang, the most intense dose of adrenalin hit me. Focused, I was back at it. Big breath, 1000, 2000... Another big breath. This happened several more times.

Then all of a sudden, my husband regained consciousness, taking a deep breath. Just like that, like a miracle had just occurred. The first thing my husband said to me was, "You look stressed". I was. He would later talk of having a white light experience.

After many tests, we learned my husband had a previously unknown congenital heart condition causing his aorta valve to slowly calcify. Upon extreme exertion, like riding up the hill, it blocked the blood flow, causing him to have a cardiac arrest. He had open heart surgery several weeks later, where doctors replaced his valve with a mechanical valve. Unfortunately, there were complications with his heart. For nearly a year, he lived a half-life, becoming progressively exhausted as cardiologists tried to determine what was wrong.

It resulted in him being diagnosed with constrictive pericarditis. He was opened up again eighteen months after his first operation. Sadly, his heart suffered again from constrictive pericarditis, which is very rare. He once again, for the third time, required more heart surgery, which took place eighteen months after his second operation.

Ironically, two days before my husband was admitted into hospital for surgery, his mother whom we lived with, also had a heart attack and was taken to hospital by ambulance. Mother and son spent Christmas in the cardiac ward, one room apart from each other.

After the initial trauma of my husband's cardiac arrest, stressed out, I lost 12kg in three weeks. Throughout this time, seeing him slowly go down-hill health wise and becoming very depressed, I feared he would have another heart attack and die.

I suffered from depression and anxiety, and while I took antidepressant medication, I sought little help except for short periods of counselling. I limited my social engagements and gave up my career as a journalist with a high-profile newspaper to become my husband's carer. I assisted him in his career as a television cameraman, until he could no longer work. For me, this has been the most challenging period of my life so far. It is hard seeing a loved one chronically ill, in pain and suffering, especially while he is trying to do basic things like get out of bed and walk from one room to another.

I felt I was a horrible person because there was a part of me that desperately wanted to run away from all of this, and I imagined everyone else having a fun time while I felt stuck. I wished he would get better.

Six months after his third heart operation, once he was well, I decided to leave my husband and returned home to my family in Australia –

where I could get help and relax. I had already had a problem with anxiety. I would get scared about making mistakes, despite being told repeatedly that everyone does, and with a positive attitude I could look upon them as learning opportunities.

I freaked out about socialising, having to walk up and talk to strangers – I hid in bed fretting about my past and my future. I did not want to face a soul. I worried that my friends and family didn't like me, that I would be abandoned and that I couldn't live up to people's expectations of me. I thought I was hopeless. I felt terribly guilty for leaving my husband.

Stressed beyond measure, I was called to a family emergency, which would show just how strained I really was. My stress was reignited again by my grandma having a fall for which she was rushed to hospital, diagnosed with multiple mini-strokes.

In the ambulance and on her way, I walked back into the house. I had a tight, burning feeling across my chest, which resembled the sensation I had experienced before while having a panic attack. I can remember momentarily thinking, *here we go again*, going back in my mind to caring for my husband, when I felt the most painful feeling in my chest. I took two steps and slid down the wall. It was the worst feeling I have ever experienced; sweating and exhausted, my body felt like it had been hit by a truck. I lay in the foetal position on a cold tiled floor in the middle of winter, unable to move.

My mother called for another ambulance. In hospital, tests concluded I had had a heart attack. I was thirty-four years old. Further tests led doctors to diagnose it as stress induced, brought on by a large dose of adrenalin which closed an artery in my heart.

From that point on, I started listening to my body; not the constant, endless chatter of my worried mind. I received help from the cardiac care clinic. On their recommendation, I benefited from monitored exercise, whole nutrition, physiotherapy, stress management, psychological counselling, yoga, and meditation.

While I would never wish this on anyone, having experienced it all has made me a stronger person. I found courage and with it, a strength I did not know I had. There is no doubt in my mind that this experience has changed me.

It has been humbling. I have learnt more than I wanted to know about fear, anxiety and desperation. I know now that I should have spent time looking after myself first. I thought, "If he is happy, I will be happy," except ill people are rarely happy. I know now to ask for help, and not pretend everything is okay – until breaking point.

I have also learnt what is most important to me: having a healthy mind, body and spirit, finding joy in simple things, living in the present moment, and truly loving myself (with all my faults) and appreciating the connection I share with friends and family.

My biggest lesson has come in understanding that I have no control over what happens, but I can manage my reaction to it. I just wish I had not learnt this the hard way. I shall take this opportunity to thank my friends and family for their love and support over the last five years. I am most grateful to you for reminding me things would get better, when I wasn't so sure.

The following information is written by experts in their fields. This may help empower you to manage your own health which will ultimately impact how you live your life.

AROMATHERAPY

How Aromatherapy Works

Essential oils have been used for over 4,000 years as medicine and also for pleasure. They are highly valued in the Eastern cultures including the Middle East, India, Egypt and China. Ayurveda, the art of Indian Healing, has used oils for thousands of years for healing and rejuvenating purposes.

When an essential oil is inhaled, it travels through the nasal passage up to the limbic brain which is also the seat of the emotional centre, mood and memory.

Humans can only pick up the smell of about 300 different odorant receptors – dogs have many more. These odorant molecules are converted to electrical impulses which travel to the limbic system. When you smell an essential oil that is utilised for its calming effect, the hypothalamus receives the input to relax, and it creates neuro-chemicals that are sent through the body to relax and calm. Likewise, an essential oil used as a stimulus, when inhaled, awakens the limbic system which will send a message of euphoria and a message to the body to energise.

Smells considered pleasant have a beneficial effect on your mood, whereas smells that are unpleasant can have a detrimental effect on your mental wellbeing.

- *Aromatic baths are relaxing and soothing, always add the essential oil at the last minute as oils evaporate quickly.*
- *Aromatic massage is a wonderful way to incorporate the oils into your body; this can be stimulating, relaxing or detoxifying depending on the massage.*
- *Adding drops to creams and lotions make for a pleasant fragrance for your personal beauty needs.*
- *Adding oils to an oil burner sends an aroma throughout the home.*

Using Essential Oils Safely

NEVER TAKE ESSENTIAL OILS BY MOUTH

- Store oils in a cool place out of children's reach. Keep oils away from eyes.
- No more than six drops of oil in the bath.
- Do not use essential oils in pregnancy unless under professional advice (NOT in the first three months as there is a risk of miscarriage).
- If you suffer from epilepsy, high blood pressure or some other medical ailment, seek professional advice first.
- If currently using prescribed medication, seek professional advice as some essential oils interact with medication.
- Use essential oils with caution on babies, children and the elderly (safest oils are chamomile, rose and lavender).
- Dilute essential oils well if using on sensitive skin, keep out of the sun as they are sensitive to sunlight and may cause burning (do a patch test first on your skin to test for sensitivity).

A superior quality essential oil will be expensive and should have '100% pure' written on the label. However, it will last a long time as the oil is concentrated and can be added to other oils and creams.

The Why & How of Aromatherapy

Aromatherapy is a gift from Mother Nature to heal and nurture the body and soul. Most essential oils found in plants, flowers, leaves, fruit and seeds serve to deter insects and predators and protect against bacterial or fungal infections. Similarly, when we use essential oils provided by Mother Nature, they serve a similar purpose to defend against disease and provide protection. Aromatherapy is also used in cuisines and as medicines for good health. The aroma & properties of plants stimulates our olfactory nerves which are responsible for our sense of smell. Essential oils can stimulate or relax our mind and our mood and are also used in massage to promote the body's own natural healing ability. In a holistic approach to health and wellbeing, essential oils bring mystical, emotional and physical benefits which have been used for thousands of years.

> *Aromatherapy is a gift from Mother Nature to heal and nurture the body and soul.*

In summary, essential oils can increase your sense of well-being, can help relieve pain or stress and are also effective for minor wounds and healing.

ASTROBACH

"There is no true healing unless there is change in outlook, peace of mind and inner happiness." - P Chancellor, Handbook of Bach Flowers Remedies

Bach flowers originated in the 1930s by Doctor Edward Bach, who was a Medical Doctor, Scientist, Homoeopathist and Bacteriologist in London in 1930s.

Dr Bach also had a keen interest in the esoteric subjects, including astrology. He noticed that there were several associations between planetary positions and personality, particularly the moon as this represents the emotional nature of the person. He believed that a physical symptom of disease directly correlates to the mind and your emotions. Your emotions act through the brain, affecting the nervous/immune systems creating negative stress causing illness. His philosophy of healing was if harmony could be restored to the persons mental and emotional states, then the individual can deal with life in a positive manner. By achieving this state, you reduce stress, which causes disease. He believed there was a simple, safe, inexpensive and natural method that would bring about self-healing.

There are twelve Bach flowers and Dr. Bach linked them to the twelve zodiac signs. Astrobach are personalised blends based on the personal astrological medical chart you were born with. The Astrobach blends work on your auric/energy field.

Our energy field is our body's first line of natural protection and therefore it is our first level of immunity. Astrobach blends work on the vibrational frequency within our energy field. If taken in a time of crisis or uncertainty, Astrobach blends will give clarity, strengthen your vital energy and enhance inner harmony to support through times of stress.

Bach Flowers originate from plants picked at certain cycles, water found in springs known for its curative properties, certain trees, bushes and from the grain family. These remedies are designed to treat to treat the whole person, not just the symptoms. Full effects of the treatment take 7-14 days.

Bach Flowers can be used:
- To relieve mental and emotional states.
- Preventatively or acutely.
- In conjunction with medicines.
- On pets, children and while pregnant.
- In combination with other natural therapies.
- Can help with depression, grief and transition.
- On plants.

Rachel Wright Naturopath, Christina Richter R.N. Health Astrologer
www.theherbary.co.nz, www.christinarichterauthor.com

BOWEN THERAPY

Bowen is a unique noninvasive soft tissue therapy that has profound effects on various chronic disorders. These include degenerated spine, arthritis, rheumatism, stress, chronic fatigue, acidity, fractures, sprains, sports injuries, muscular skeletal disorders, asthma, and nervous disorders. It is also beneficial in maintaining mental and emotional equilibrium, as well as 'women's problems' including fertility and other associated conditions.

An Australian, Tom Bowen, initiated this therapy (which is named after him) and since its inception, has been taught worldwide by the Bowen Therapy Founders, Oswald and Elaine Rentsch.

> *...sometimes it is known as homeopathy of bodywork...*

Sometimes it is known as homeopathy of bodywork. Bowen Therapy utilises small, but measured inputs to the body, stimulating the body to heal itself, often profoundly. The Bowen technique is unique in that it offers tremendous benefit to clients with very little effort on the part of the practitioner.

The Bowen technique addresses the entire body by restoring balance via the Autonomic Nervous System (ANS), rather than focusing on a single complaint. The ANS controls over 80% of body functions and is very susceptible to external stressors. In today's world, most people live in a constant state of high stress and sympathetic ANS over-stimulation, fight, flight or freeze mode. Healing can occur only after the ANS shifts from sympathetic to parasympathetic dominance, rest, relax and repair mode.

The Bowen technique seems to be the catalyst that influences this to happen. The common observation is that Bowen sessions seem to reactivate the recovery process in situations where healing from trauma, sickness or surgery has stalled or reached a plateau.

In Bowen Therapy, specific moves are made on ligaments, tendons or muscles which most likely activate the Golgi receptors and send signals to the brain, the neurological pathways, the fascia, also activating the meridians, and the electromagnetic field of the person.

Bowen also assists in balancing the elements and the Doshas from the Ayurvedic perspective. That is why Prof Dr. P.H. Kulkarni calls it a 'Marma Chikitsa'.

Firadia Irania www.subtleenergies.co.nz

DEPRESSION

My Journey with Depression

How did I know there was something wrong?
I am a forty-five-year-old, very busy wife and mother with three children; one with a disability. I worked a full-time job in part time hours. I am married to a self-employed electrician running his own business. I knew there was something wrong with me when I started to find it very difficult to get out of bed in the morning. Initially, I didn't really feel well physically. I thought that maybe I had the flu, or a cold, or maybe I was just tired. I took time off work to recover from these physical ailments, but found that with each day, I just felt worse. It was very hard to try to describe my feelings to my husband or other members of my family and friends.

To give you some examples, I found the simplest things overwhelming. I would feel panicked about going to the supermarket. It would take a long time to have a shower and get dressed in the morning. I found simple tasks difficult to finish. I can remember thinking that tidying up the kitchen was a huge task. I wanted nothing to do with technology. Cell phones, texting, emails and Facebook became my enemies. It was unusual for me, being a people person, not to want to talk to anyone. So, I knew there was something very wrong.

How did it affect my mind, thinking, health and family?
I started to read about depression. It is not good to self-diagnose, but I was pretty sure about it, as I had most of the symptoms. I felt like I was down a dark hole, and I could not dig myself out. I did not want to go to the doctor, because I knew he would prescribe medication, and I did not want to be 'one of those people'.

This all happened at a time when my young son had just come out of hospital, had both legs in plaster, was completely immobile, and needed a wheel chair to get around. I was supposed to be the one in charge of his primary care, which was a problem at the time, as I could not even look after myself. My husband found this difficult to understand, because I looked fine. As there was nothing visibly and/or physically wrong with me, it was hard for him to comprehend, as there was nothing for him to physically fix. He was angry and was also emotionally affected by what was happening to me. He didn't know how to deal with me. The children knew there was something wrong, because I was not acting like myself. The structure of our family life started to crumble, and my husband wasn't coping with it.

My mind felt like jelly. I could only think about one thing at a time. I am used to thinking about ten things at a time. My house looked awful. I couldn't get out of my dressing gown.

What did I do?
Thank God for my sister who rang me at the right time and told me to go down to the doctor to get on some medication. Although she is a fan of natural therapies, she knew that I had gone past the point of no return. Once you are past that point, sometimes you do need proper medical intervention to get your equilibrium back. You need to bring yourself back to a point

where you can then be receptive to further help, through natural therapies. When I knew there was something wrong, I did go to an acupuncturist, but really, this didn't even touch the sides.

Medical intervention
The antidepressants have helped me enormously. I can now function, whereas before, I couldn't get out of bed. As my son was in plaster, it was important for me to do all the normal things: get out of bed, give everyone their breakfast, make their lunch, take the kids to school, clean the house, make dinner and deal with after school activities; in other words, function normally. I could not do any of those things prior to going to my doctor. I was not functioning on any level. However, within two weeks of taking the medication the doctor prescribed, I was back on a bit more of an even keel. Then my sister came over for a week and recommended some natural therapies.

Natural and other therapies
One of the nicest things that I did for myself was to experience energy healing. My understanding of it is limited, however, I think how it works is that the energy healer works to unblock areas of your body where energy is low, or energy is stuck.

I lay down on a table and listened to some quiet music while the energy healing was being performed on me. During the experience, it was very relaxing. I could see quite vivid colours in my 'mind's eye'. I saw many colours, including purple, yellow and white. In terms of its immediate effects, I felt very relaxed and peaceful. At the end of the session, I 'awoke' feeling refreshed. I don't know how it works. I just know that it does. In terms of the longer-term effects, the energy healings helped 'lift the fog' from my brain. I feel there is a direct connection between the energy healings and my increased energy levels. I felt a lot more focused, and more able to concentrate, and deal with the functional elements of living.

I have been doing many other things to bring back balance into my life. I took on board a comprehensive vitamin regime to 'top up' on those areas where I had depleted my resources. I have also been walking on the beach, near the sea, taking in some sun, and listening to meditation CD's which I find very soothing.

The connection between medical therapy and natural therapy
In many ways, being on the medication gave me the ability to then take on board the natural therapies that my sister recommended. I do really feel that traditional medicine and natural medicine have worked together to give me the best possible result.

How do I feel now?
I feel great! I am functioning like a normal human being. I am back into a full-time role, which I am really enjoying.

My life is still very busy, and I don't believe that will ever change. However, some things have changed. I realise now that it is important to make time for myself, to do things that are nurturing for me, which have nothing to do with my husband, children, or friends. I know I need to make time for exercise, as this is a great way to clear my head. I know that, sometimes, I need to put myself first, which is something I am not used to doing. I now know that, sometimes, I need to say 'no' to friends and family. This is something I have never done before.

I am trying to stop and smell the roses a bit more! It's a fine balancing act, or put another way, a continual work in progress!

Anonymous

Treating Depression Naturally

Depression is becoming an ever-increasing problem in today's world. Almost every person is stressed for a variety of reasons. Some people have strategies in place in their lives to reduce this pressure, but many do not. Just simple steps can be beneficial in maintaining a healthy state of mind as suggested below:

- St. John's Wort (Hypericum) is uplifting, though can take up to ten days to start showing any results. *Contraindicated in lactation and may interact with oral contraception and some prescribed medications: check with your doctor.*
- Ginger, fennel, cumin, fenugreek, peppers all beneficial to stimulate metabolism.
- Valerian, chamomile, sleepy time tea, warm milk with nutmeg or cinnamon to assist with sleeping problems.
- Increase intake of raw fruits and vegetables, cereals, green leafy vegetables and whole grains.
- Decrease consumption of dairy and fat.
- Remove stimulants such as coffee and coca cola – replace with herbal teas.
- Mango, passion fruit, seafood, Brazil nuts and spinach are natural mood elevators.
- Increase intake of vitamin B especially B2, B6, magnesium, zinc and vitamin C.
- Boost consumption of fish oils and omega-3s.
- Grains, chicken, turkey, soybeans, organic honey, peas, and liquorice are natural antidepressants.
- Magnet therapy can also be of assistance.
- Acupuncture has been successfully used for relaxation for hundreds of years.
- Avoid wearing black, blue, browns or dark colours as they depress the immune system.
- Wear light colours only, green, yellow, reds, orange, purples, pinks and white.

- Walk barefoot on grass or beach, as often as possible. This is also good for grounding.
- Spend as much time as possible in the sunshine on a regular basis.
- Allow time each day to exercise or walk as much as possible, as well as deep breathing.
- Aromatherapy oils such as orange, rose, geranium, lavender (or bergamot in a burner) are great in the bath or in massage oils.
- Listen to upbeat music, not only can music provide a calming effect, but it is positive as well.
- Monitor your thoughts - catch negative thoughts and change to positive ones.
- Use positive affirmations.
- Sing loudly and frequently.
- Discuss your feelings and thoughts with someone you trust.
- Cry, rather than bottle up your emotions, as this releases blocks.
- Keep a diary and be creative, paint, dance, or draw. Creativity increases your self-esteem which promotes a positive attitude.
- Watch comedy on television or at the movies. Read amusing literature (i.e. jokes) laugh and try and mix with happy light-hearted people, chose your friends carefully.

GESTALT THERAPY OR VOICE DIALOGUE

For an in-depth understanding of all the implications of Gestalt Therapy, a three-year programme is usually completed, so it is a psychotherapy degree in its own right. However, it can also be very useful in quite a simple form and is quick and immediate in consultation work. Gestalt Therapy was developed by Frederick Perls in the 1960s from much older material; all his books are wonderfully insightful and fascinating. Voice Dialogue arises from the Gestalt Model and was developed by Hal Stone.

Perl's key concept involved his belief that many personalities lack wholeness and are fragmented. He claims that people are only aware of parts of themselves, rather than the whole self. Gestalt Therapy involves a dialogue between the fragmented selves, so the whole person may get to know the individual parts of the whole, leading to increased awareness.

We link this with another model known as 'psycho-synthesis' from Roberto Assagioli, also in the 1960s. Sub-personalities, known as 'voices', are encouraged to become aware of each other, and accept their distinct roles in the 'whole person'. Once this occurs, the potential for synthesis between the voices is possible, as they learn to work together toward the potential for every individual person.

> ...He claims that people are only aware of parts of themselves rather than the whole self...

We have many 'voices' or characters within our psyche. These are the key to the psycho-emotional transactions at play within the psyche, and therefore lead to our behaviours and outcomes at any given moment. All voices are 'good', not 'bad' - even though they may be causing trouble! Rather, they are either functional or dysfunctional in terms of these outcomes. Our 'voices' contain our core unconscious beliefs about our right to be happy, successful, useful, free to welcome change, responsible, smart... and so on. These were programmed between birth and the age of seven in the early family system.

In adult life, our 'voices' play out their core beliefs - some positive and functional and others limiting, thus dysfunctional. They set up 'games' and conflict within our psyche and in our outer world, because they are at odds with each other in their attempts to get their needs met.

The voices play out externally by 'dreaming up' people to express one end of the voice 'split' - hence relationships and family areas are where we meet our 'Soul Pod' and play out our Karmic Cauldron process - our greatest tests and lessons. Limiting voices contain the growth potential of the lifetime, because we unconsciously repeat these patterns until we've learnt our lesson and achieve our soul growth. Once we learn the lesson contained in these patterns, then they may begin to resolve into functional potential - this is the 'Alchemical Gold'.

Once the voices learn to honour and hear each other, then their stress is released into constructive mutual antagonism. Limiting voices never go away, however our journey requires consciously learning to manage and understand these facets of our psychological makeup and learn to make the best of them!

Gestalt Therapy is a valuable tool in unlocking the dynamics of our limiting 'voices' as this offers a simple and practical method of meeting our inner voices, and finding out how they feel about each other, and why they are maintaining certain positions of belief with resultant behaviours.

I usually offer my clients this option quite spontaneously during a session, when we have reached a point of clarifying that there is some stress in how the client is experiencing a particular feature of their makeup. So, perhaps we have identified that he/she has a voice that wants to stay home and be very responsible and organised - and probably organise the whole family to within an inch of their lives!

Meanwhile, a second voice is hugely outgoing and social, and very dynamic in business and with social/people issues. Obviously, they are going to have a problem dealing with each other, until they learn to see that both of their positions are absolutely okay and valid, and that they are potentially very good for each other!

One possible expression here is that they have a partner who is externalised in the world, and they are doing the anchoring at home, but feeling very put upon by all that they do, and letting the partner know about this - "I work so hard and you have so much fun - it's not fair!" It is not hard to see from this example that these two inner characters are going to feel very differently, and that a dialogue between them could be most revealing.

As the facilitator, you will sit in a chair in front of two empty chairs, which are placed next to each other, and facing each other at a slight angle. This enables the most non-threatening position for the two voices who will be talking to each other.

Gestalt Therapy is a valuable tool in unlocking the dynamics of our limiting 'voices'...

Invite the client to sit in one of the chairs and introduce yourself to the voice and tell it a little about who it is, so they can begin to get in touch with this inner character. For instance: "Hello Mrs Responsible, it's great to meet you. I know you are a very hard-working gal who does quite a bit of taking care of others and being responsible." Allow her to respond and go from there....

The trick with Gestalt is to watch and listen to what is unfolding - body language, tone of voice, demeanour, attitude and so on - and go with it. Is it happy, sad, hostile, frightened, serious, frivolous etc.? This leads you - they do their own revealing - all you need to do is nurture and give permission for the voice to fully express itself.

If your intuition tells you that another voice is emerging, or you feel that voice one has finished stating its position, then find the appropriate point to complete with voice one and tell it that you will come back and talk again later. Invite the client to change chairs and continue the process.

Be humorous - be relaxed - enjoy what is happening so they can too!

Emotions emerge quite quickly I find, so go with them and support them. Here you will need some basic client-centred counselling skills, lots of compassion, and your own honest ability to 'name the drama' which they are revealing to themselves. Classic phrases like, "it sounds like you are... exhausted, frightened, anxious, nervous"; "how does... make you feel?"; "I guess that makes you feel pretty... angry, sad, frightened etc."; "my fantasy about this part of you is that he/she would really like to...."

The typical revelation which emerges out of a dialogue between two voices, is that one of them is holding the 'goodie' position, whilst the other is being set up to hold the 'baddie' position. Conflict resolution is the goal here. The

> *Conflict resolution is the goal here.*

two voices must be encouraged to hear and understand the other's position, which in turn can lead to understanding, softening and forgiveness. As you are talking with each voice and information is emerging, invite the voice to name itself - sometimes a silly name - absolutely anything goes here.

Usually the voice that has been 'in control' (usually perceived as the 'bad' voice) has been protecting something deep within that is vulnerable or hurt or angry or frightened. Part of your job is to validate this and commend the voice for all the work it has done during life to keep protecting, and that it is okay to stop doing this in quite the same way. In other words, it is time to 'get safe' enough to let this voice go off duty! The process is about negotiation between the two (or sometimes more) voices. This is often very tenuous, so your words can be along these lines: "Are you willing to allow your other voice (name) to...? If he/she agrees to..., what do you need in return?"

Then, change chairs and go back and do the other voice. So, follow through here with: "Did you hear what he/she offered? Are you willing to trust this? Do you need any guarantees?"

I find that in many situations one of the voices is frightened that the other voice is 'risky' in some way, and they are afraid that if they let out this other potentially risky character, something awful might happen. So, the question becomes: "What might happen if you let him/her have more room to express him/herself (or get out of the cupboard, as I call it)?"

Sometimes the Gestalt process can become quite complex if you keep inviting other voices to get in on the act. The whole trick is to keep track of all the relationships with each other and attempt to bring about resolution between what usually turns out to be the two main teams: the strong team versus the sensitive team - strong versus weak: the archetypal essence of the 'whole person' process.

I usually recommend that once the client has named their voices and is more aware of their needs and wants, then they can simply learn to 'talk to themselves' whenever they need to clear or unblock an inner tension or confusion. Be your own therapist!

Once we become aware of our 'stuck bits' and learn to unblock them in these simple, effective and enlightening ways, it is amazing how quickly we remove stress from our lives and begin to feel more balanced and whole!

www.universalastrology.com.au © Maggie Kerr

HOMEOPATHY

A young boy came to me with a huge fear of waking in the night, thinking of scary things. He doesn't like to go to the bathroom by himself when it is dark. He is even afraid of toys with smiley faces. His mother is getting tired of having disturbed sleep. For some children, the exploration of the world outside their family can be a scary experience and parents may observe the child starts regressing to baby-ish behaviours.

Visiting a homeopath is a quiet, safe place for a child to talk about how they are feeling. I have noticed children busy playing with toys will usually have one ear on the conversation between parent and the homeopath, and a confident child will butt in if the story isn't quite right. A

> *Visiting a homeopath is a quiet safe place for a child to talk about how they are feeling.*

less confident child runs to mum or dad for snuggles, seeking protection and reassurance that they are still loved.

A well indicated homeopathic medicine can help the child make the transition to kindergarten or school more easily and opens the way for parents to understand more about the family dynamic. Is there jealousy or bullying between siblings going on at home or school?

In recent years, homeopathic medicines have been made from human substances (e.g. breast milk, placental tissue, umbilical cord) and these can be very useful for children who long to return to the safety of the womb or have not been able to separate from mum in a healthy way. A traumatic birth or uterine deficiency may indicate the need for these human medicines. The homeopathic medicines are highly diluted in water and safe to take at any age. Parents notice their child confidently spends time at kindergarten or school after these homeopathic medicines. They settle more easily at night and often the fears disappear just as quickly as they came.

Angela Hair is a homeopath from Hastings with twenty years' experience.

Contact her through concordiahealth.co.nz website or text 02 7443 6737

MĀORI HEALING

In the Māori culture, the Tohunga (priest/priestess) defines *romiromi* as a philosophy of life that links and channels the energies of timeless spiritual phenomena of nature. The Māori takutaku (prescriptive healing chants to the spiritual phenomena of nature) are instrumental in clearing spiritual entities and shifting unwanted energies held in the cellular memory of the body. Using wood, plants, greenstone, sound, earth, water and intuitive diagnosis, the rituals and practices of romiromi are used to unblock and release spiritual, physical, emotional, mental and generational trauma.

My recent doctoral research sought to validate indigenous forms of romiromi healing, revealing ancient mother epistemologies of nature i.e., Papatūānuku (earth mother), Hinemarama (Grandmother of the Moon), Hinemoana-nui (Grandmother of the Ocean), Hine-nui-te-po (Grandmother of the stardust) to name but a few, as the source of healing for families. My research findings validated the existence of divine feminine beings in various forms of oral Māori literature, including waiata (songs), karakia (incantations to nature), takutaku (healing chants to nature), moteatea (chants that tell the local history), whakataukī (proverbs) and pūrākau (stories).

Positive holistic health outcomes were identified for Māori families in my research when the philosophies, rituals and practices of romiromi healing were being normalised into everyday family life. As a result, the transmission of healing knowledge was instrumental in the kaitiakitanga (guardianship) of Papatūānuku mother-nature and her progeny. The philosophy of reciprocity in this context, being that in healing mother earth and her progeny, we in turn receive healing. Manu Korewha, a Ngaapuhi Tohunga Ahurewa (priest of a higher order), proposes to heal the mother and you will heal the entire family.

> *Positive holistic health outcomes were identified for Maori families in my research...*

I currently work as a lecturer of mātauranga Māori in early childhood education but have also been a cultural bodyworker for over twenty years, as well as a contemporary Te Oomai Reia romiromi, Māori healing practitioner, for over a decade. As a research project manager in local Māori health research in Hawkes Bay and a Director for the Harata Meretana Ma

Charitable Trust, I continue to coordinate and facilitate national Māori healing romiromi wānanga (intergenerational learning on a marae setting) in low socio-economic Māori communities. Using the philosophy of romiromi in my work extends to professional supervision for mental health workers. I also mentor mental health whai-ora to get to the core of spiritual imbalance, thus empowering them to take back their own power and live to their full potential.

Naku Noa Na Charlotte Mildon www.aiohealing.com Ph: 027 557 5002
© Copyright 8 August 2016

MASSAGE

Massage – what you don't know

Most people frequent massage clinics on a regular basis. Whether it is just a quick thirty-minute foot rub, a break from shopping, or an all over body pamper to erase weekly accumulated stress, massage can be of benefit in any situation.

Massage is one of the most ancient forms of healing. The first writings on massage appeared around 2000 BC. The ancient Greeks and Romans used massage to obtain and maintain good health and promote healing. Unfortunately, today, massage is usually seen as a treat, or a last resort: "I need a massage, my back is killing me." While it is a popular form of healing, the average person is missing the holistic benefits this ancient art can provide. Massage used correctly can restore balance to the emotional and physical wellbeing of its users.

Massage is one of the most ancient forms of healing.

Massage may appear to merely be a lot of pressing and 'feel-good' kneading on the skin, but it is actually a scientific process. Therapeutic touch stimulates the release of endorphins, the body's natural pain killer, inducing a feeling of wellbeing. This assists in relaxation and reduced levels of stress hormones, such as cortisol and noradrenaline, which weaken the immune system. Massage will in fact, increase the healthy functioning of every organ in your body!

Massage also increases your blood flow and lymph circulation. Lymph is a fluid that rids the body tissues of waste and is dependent on the squeezing/milking effects of the muscles. For people who undertake regular exercise, their lymph flow will be good, but those with an inactive lifestyle will have sluggish bodies with stagnant waste products. The human lymph system is vital to our life force; if these toxins and waste are not removed from the body, they will create blockages.

Massage dramatically aids lymph movement, which, together with blood, supplies nutrients and oxygen and rids the body of waste and toxins. Good circulation is so important for health, and massage can be so beneficial for this purpose. This milking action by the muscles metabolically maintains a chemical balance within the body. However, this balance will only be maintained through normal activity.

If you are over-active, you are not allowing the body sufficient relaxation time for the inflow of nutrient products to feed your body and assist in the removal of toxins. As a result, toxic products are formed faster than can be eliminated and, consequently, muscles will be loaded with irritant acids. Similarly, under-activity will not provide this milking effect by the muscles to assist lymph and venous return. In this situation, toxins formed within tissues will not be carried away and will sit in the same spot until some physical activity occurs.

Toxin build up within the body will affect wellbeing dramatically, resulting in feelings of lethargy, and possibly, depression. Muscles will become inactive, affecting the surrounding structures which will limit the range of movement resulting in pain and discomfort.

Stress is another major factor affecting everybody's life. We feel the effect of stress, but we rarely notice what long-term impact it has on our mental and physical wellbeing. Each thought that enters our head creates a vibration; it is estimated that our brains produce as many as 12,000 to 50,000 thoughts per day depending on how 'deep' a thinker we are - that's a lot of thoughts! However, this will not be a surprise to those who meditate. People who meditate are familiar with the Havoc Mind Phenomenon in which the mind is observed as an out-of-control thought generator.

In regular life, the disturbing aspect of these 50,000 thoughts per day is that the vast majority of them are pure nonsense. Our thinking often dwells in the past or the future, obsessing about mistakes we might have made, battling guilt, planning or worrying. Our thoughts constantly drift in and out of fantasy, fiction and negativity, resulting in unnoticed negative vibrations, so it becomes almost 'normal' to feel this way.

However, vibrations don't come and go the same way thoughts do. These vibrations will gather together and become embedded in your energy field. Long-term bottled up energy from negative thought patterns and suppressed issues, will eventually explode in your aura. When your body becomes overloaded with these vibrations, this will lead to disease, illness and if not resolved, death.

> *Long term bottled up energy, from negative thought patterns and suppressed issues, will eventually explode in your aura.*

The body is a highly intelligent machine. If shown something, it will remember it, even if on a conscious level you yourself don't know has occurred. So, by receiving regular massage, allowing the body to see a new state of balance and ease, it will recognise this and through repetition, this desired state will become a natural habit.

Every human being experiences some form of stress, whether through work, family, environment or society. Mental tension, frustrations and insecurities cause the most damage. Hormones released by stress shrink blood vessels, inhibiting circulation. A stressed mind and body means the heart works harder, breathing becomes rapid and shallow and digestion slows. Almost every body process is degraded. Massage can amazingly counteract the effects of stress.

The benefits of massage on a weekly to fortnightly basis are extremely beneficial. It can keep you healthy, remove toxins including cellulite, help slow down the aging process, normalise your hormones, tone the body and provide a sense of peace and calm for mind and body alike.

The most important thing to consider when commencing massage as a regular and vital part of your life regime, is to make sure you find a good massage therapist. Research thoroughly and seek recommendations from friends and associates. There are a lot of frauds in this industry who will only provide a 'feel good' massage and not the 'holistic massage' properly trained masseurs can provide.

Amalie Cardile: Amalie Day Spa

www.facebook.com/AmaliaDaySpa

MEDITATION

"Meditation is the expression of the intelligence that links life and form, the self and the not-self in time and in the three worlds. The process of this connection eventuates on the plane of mind, which links the higher and the lower." – Prof Dr. P H Kulkarni

When we think of meditation, we often envisage the ancient Yogis sitting in the lotus position and chanting mantras, or focusing on nothing, without thought, reaching the sublime state of blankness where the emphasis is on the space between the in-breath and the out-breath. We then believe that meditation is difficult, requiring years of dedicated training and practice. While this may be true for the above-mentioned forms of meditation, and the dedication is well worth it, there are other forms of meditation which are so simple that anyone can achieve them.

> *...there are forms of meditation which are so simple that anyone can achieve them.*

Have you ever had a daydream where your thoughts wandered off to somewhere beautiful, where you were blissfully unaware of your actual surroundings until interrupted? You were in a state of meditation.

Have you ever been focusing so intently on what you were doing that you lost track of time or didn't notice someone come into the room? Again, this is another example of meditation. What about suddenly seeing something stunningly beautiful that causes you to inhale and exhale deeply, that kind of "Wow!" Yes, you guessed it, meditation. The hypnogogic meditative state, what elite athletes call 'the zone', is also reached through martial arts, dance, art, music, drumming, chanting, yoga, and tai chi, to name but a few.

Meditative disciplines encompass a wide range of goals from simply a more relaxed and peaceful frame of mind, increased creativity or self-awareness, compassion and loving kindness, to achieving a higher state of consciousness or enlightenment. The practice of meditation enables your thoughts to be calm and clear, thereby increasing your mental capacity and facilitating your decision making. The ability to focus your attention, to concentrate, is enhanced. Memory is improved, learning and assimilating new knowledge becomes easier.

Thereby, your attribute of self-respect grows, giving you inner strength, to follow your own potential and be all that you can be, bringing true tranquility. Intuition becomes activated and strengthened and you find it easier to manage situations that life places before you.

Though meditation is largely recognised as a spiritual practice, it also has many health benefits. Practicing meditation has positive effects on physical and mental health and wellbeing. Yoga and meditation techniques are being implemented in the management of life threatening diseases; in transformation of molecular and genetic structure; in reversal of mental illnesses; in accelerated learning programs; in perceptions and communications beyond the physical; in solving problems; in atomic and nuclear physics; in gaining better ecological understanding and in management of lifestyle.

> *Though meditation is largely recognised as a spiritual practice, it also has many health benefits.*

Some of the physical benefits of regular meditation are:

- Deep rest - as measured by decreased metabolic rate, lower heart rate, and reduced work load of the heart.

- Lowered levels of cortisol and lactate - two chemicals associated with stress.
- Reduction of free radicals, which are unstable oxygen molecules that can cause tissue damage. They are now thought to be a major factor in aging and in many diseases.
- Decreased high blood pressure.
- Raises skin resistance as low skin resistance is correlated with higher stress and anxiety levels.
- Drop in cholesterol levels. High cholesterol is associated with cardiovascular disease.
- Improved flow of air to the lungs resulting in easier breathing. This has been very helpful to asthma patients.
- Younger biological age. On standard measures of aging, long-term Meditation practitioners measured up to 12 years younger than their chronological age.
- Higher levels of DHEAS in the elderly. An additional sign of youthfulness through Meditation; lower levels of DHEAS are associated with aging.
- It lowers oxygen consumption and decreases respiratory rate.
- It increases blood flow and slows the heart rate.
- Increases exercise tolerance in heart patients.
- Leads to a deeper level of relaxation.
- Decreases muscle tension and headaches.
- Builds self-confidence.
- It increases serotonin production which influences mood and behaviour. Low levels of serotonin are associated with depression, obesity, insomnia and headaches.
- Helps in chronic diseases like allergies, arthritis etc.
- Reduces Pre-menstrual Syndrome.

- Helps in post-operative healing.
- Enhances the immune system. Research has revealed that meditation increases activity of the body's natural cells, which kill bacteria and cancer cells.
- Reduces activity of viruses and emotional distress.

In my personal experience, I have also found meditation to be a highly effective tool in pain management and pain cessation.

One part of this life's journey was for me to experience firsthand the effects of breast cancer and its spread. In 2006, it had progressed to the point where I was diagnosed with an incurable tumor in my right axilla (underarm). The tumor had infiltrated the brachial plexus nerve and artery and was causing extreme pain which required 150-200 mg of slow release morphine plus frequent 'breakthrough' doses of liquid morphine per day just to make it bearable. Whilst undergoing treatment I was even too ill to think, often wavering between consciousness and unconsciousness, particularly during times of extreme body temperature fluctuations with accompanying nausea, dizziness etc. During periods of lucidity, simple meditations and guided meditations helped me through.

After many months of intensive chemotherapy, the tumor had shrunk from 3 x 4 x 5 cm, to 2 x 3 x 4 cm but was still causing severe pain. The side effects of taking the morphine and other medications were to me, becoming intolerable.

I decided to ditch the painkillers; they were causing too many problems for too little benefit. It was during this time that I began meditating with the purpose of relieving the pain. At first all I could manage was to breathe slowly while silently saying, "There is no pain," repeatedly, and allowing the pain to leave. I did this whenever the pain became worse and slowly the pain began to lessen. After that, I altered my mantra to, "There is no pain, there is no cause for pain," believing that if meditation could remove pain, it could remove the cause.

Jennabeth Moss

MINDFULNESS

I have believed for some time that medication does not have to be the answer and that through positive thinking and trust, the body will heal and care for itself.

> ...through positive thinking and trust, the body will heal and care for itself.

I had an opportunity to 'walk my talk' so to speak, when I took my first trip to India in 2009. I was advised by friends/medical practitioners alike that I should be vaccinated and take the appropriate medical preparations for my trip. However, my intuition told me that medication was not the only option.

I felt strongly that if I believed wholeheartedly that I did not require any medical intervention to be 'protected', and if I held only positive thoughts about my health before and during the trip, that I would maintain my usual good health. I made a conscious decision not to have the vaccines and I did not allow any negative or fear-based reactions to affect me. I was also adamant that I would not get the formidable 'Delhi Belly' which is the 'inevitable' stomach bug that every traveller endures when they go to India.

I set off for a month in India and every day I acknowledged to myself that I was well and protected. Obviously, I did take small precautions like using hand sanitiser before and after food and when on trains. I also ensured that I did not eat anything raw that may have been in contact with local water. Other than this, I took no other precautions and made sure that I held strong in my belief that I was well and would be well for my entire trip. The end of my month in India arrived and I was in better health than I had been before I left. For anyone who is wondering... yes, I even managed to escape the dreaded 'Delhi Belly'. What I have taken from this is an even stronger belief that our thoughts contribute a lot to our health and that if we believe we are well, the body will look after itself without medication.

NATUROPATHIC MEDICINE

Medical naturopaths complete not only a medical degree, but also naturopathic/herbal/nutritional diplomas. Naturopathy has evolved from the ancient healing traditions of Europe. Its roots are firmly grounded in early Greek medical philosophy, but with an expanded and scientific understanding from more modern sources. Naturopathy is now recognised by mainstream medicine as a valuable and effective treatment for a variety of many diseases and disorders.

> *Naturopathy has a strong focus on the prevention of health problems and the early detection of a person's likelihood of developing a specific health problem or predisposition.*

Naturopathy has a strong focus on the prevention of health problems and the early detection of a person's likelihood of developing a specific health problem or predisposition. It is very effective at treating acute and chronic health issues because it treats the whole body, addressing all mental, and emotional aspects.

Naturopathy aims to:

- Minimise acute symptoms.
- Support the body's vital force - the capacity to self-heal.
- Re-balance the system so that illness is less likely to reoccur.
- Educate the patient to monitor their own health and the health of their family.

Naturopathy is not a single modality of healing. Today's naturopathic practitioner incorporates the most recent scientific knowledge and research with the healing wisdom of many cultures and modalities to provide a service based on the long-held principles of naturopathic medicine, which are:

- Treat the cause, rather than the effect – the underlying cause of a disease is sought and treated, not just the symptoms.
- Treat the whole person – each person is a complex interaction of mind, body and soul that can be influenced by physical, spiritual and social factors. The naturopathic practitioner will take all these factors into consideration when supporting a client.
- The healing power of nature – the naturopathic practitioner works with the body's innate ability to heal itself and facilitates this natural process with the aid of natural therapies.
- Cure without harm - by using a natural, safe and effective therapy, the naturopathic practitioner is committed to the principle of no harm.
- The physician is the teacher – the naturopathic practitioner educates, empowers and motivates clients to take responsibility for their own health.
- Prevention is the best cure – prevention of disease is accomplished through a lifestyle that supports optimal

health – Naturopathy educates clients on healthy lifestyle choices.

Naturopathic practitioners make recommendations on lifestyle and diet to produce optimal health, and in cases of disease, they combine their knowledge of natural, non-invasive healing techniques to assist nature's healing.

Dr Chris Tsioutis, MD, ND, DipNutr, DipBotMed, DipDerm, MACNEM.
Sydney Institute of Holistic & Cosmetic Medicine

PRANAYAMA

Life is held and moved around in the body with five gravity-like forces:

Apana moves it downward

Udana upward

Samana horizontally and

Vyana around the body.

Prana directs this entire dance. Prana is the conductor and the animator. Hence, out of respect, Prana is called the life force in many contexts.

When Prana is strong, life force is said to be strong and animation is harmonious.

Life appears and is experienced to be in pure health. Animation means - all normal bodily functions. For example, appetite, ability to eat, digest, absorb and eliminate are all bits of animation in the digestive system. Ability to inhale, absorb (the oxygen), eliminate all metabolic waste gases in exhalation are also animation in the respiratory system. If a function is inappropriate, then the Prana is said to be inappropriate. It could be the beginning of a health condition. Both Prana and that specific inaccurate function need to be corrected to regain health. Prana has another energetic aspect that is derived from healthy lifestyle which is behind the cellular or organic wisdom. A healthy approach to life creates energy.

> ...*a healthy approach to life creates energy...*

This energy is collected in three forms in the body:

- *Ojas*, the raw and easy-to-modify energy is the first one.
- *Tejas* is the second aspect that is responsible for attack, defense and repair.
- *Prana* is the surveillance.

Under the direction of this Prana, Tejas attacks a pathogen using Ojas energy. And Tejas rebuilds a torn tissue using Ojas.

When Prana decides to cease, animation ceases. All aspects of life cease to exist, except the decay. And it is called death.

Dealing with Prana is purely a juggling act. Unlike a typical street-side juggling, we deal with hundreds of conscious facts at the same time. This is the role of the mind. Information (or beliefs) the mind has on keeping the Prana going is exceptional. Beliefs it possesses on what's good and bad, right and wrong and comfortable and not are endless!

Mostly, we do this juggling far better than a professional juggler! Literally thousands of times better. Sometimes we get it wrong. And thus, begins the ill health.

To improve and stabilise Prana, there are many simple techniques. They are simple, because we know most of them already. We are just not convinced, that is all. Simple because most of them are inexpensive. We don't find time for them.

Here is a sample list of activities to stabilise the eight aspects of Prana. Please remember that these are just examples. Most of us might need lots of mental training to practice even these small activities.

Prana force

Exercise: slow running for 30 minutes, daily, early in the morning with appropriate dress (to sweat profusely at least for 10 minutes) and hydration.

Lifestyle: regularity - having many activities at the same time every day, such as going to bed, waking up, meals etc.

Mind: having healthy fun activities, such as group laughing.

Udana force

Exercise: climbing (rope, rock, mountain etc.) to make the body light and strong.

Lifestyle: work out tomorrow's plans today and do as much as possible to deal with them today.

Mind: finding something to apply your passion.

Samana force

Exercise: proper rest at regular intervals.

Lifestyle: applying a comfortable pace to your daily activities.

Mind: acting with equanimity, with a sense of everything (good and bad, pain and pleasure, right and wrong) is here for a reason.

Vyana force

Exercise: incorporate activities such as soccer, volleyball or cricket to use your body in various positions and roles.

Lifestyle: physically, move around daily.

Mind: try various other mentally and physically challenging activities.

Apana force

Exercise: work on your weight-bearing abilities, practice muscle toning exercises.

Prana, Tejas and Ojas energies

Do all the above in a systematic and organized way. If you have a full range of food items, physical activities etc. in a month – you are doing well. Also make sure that you are going to bed early, eating dinner early, sipping water rather than guzzling it down and chewing every mouthful thirty times!

And, the result? You wake refreshed, move your bowels two or more times a day, urinate 4-5 times a day, buzz with energy and, in short, love everything about your life.

Dr. Rama Prasad BAMS, CACH, Clinical Director at Sydney Ayurveda Centre - SydneyAyurvedaCentre.com

REBIRTHING

(Names have been changed)

Sandra awoke at 2am, drenched in sweat. Her breathing was erratic, her stomach in knots. She wanted to scream but was too afraid to make a sound. John, her husband slept soundly beside her. Sandra was in the grip of a panic she could not control or understand. Her life was sliding out of control. She had been experiencing these panic attacks for the last six months and they were becoming increasingly severe and more frequent. John would tell her to pull herself together and get over it. He could not understand why she was acting like this. In his mind, she didn't have any worries, they had been happily married for seventeen years, had two healthy children and were financially well off. Sandra also didn't understand why she was feeling this way, but her feelings were real.

A friend recommended she see me for counselling. Sandra looked distracted and tired. She was not sleeping well because she was afraid she would experience the panic attacks in her sleep, resulting in fear that stopped her from sleeping soundly. After an initial counselling consultation, I recommended we try a rebirthing breath session.

I explained to her that there are four things to remember in rebirthing. The first is the breathing: rebirthing is a dynamic breathing technique. The patient lies on a bed and breathes without pausing. This is called connected breathing.

"But won't I start to hyperventilate?" she asked. "No," I said, "hyperventilation is uncontrolled, non-voluntary and fearful, while rebirthing is controlled, voluntary and relaxed." The purpose of connected breathing is to increase the energy flow in the body by unblocking the acupuncture meridian channels.

> *The purpose of connected breathing is to increase the energy flow in the body by unblocking the acupuncture meridian channels.*

The second thing is to relax, to allow your body to be heavy, relax, inhale and exhale. Relaxing the body improves the breathing and helps the repressed emotions and memories come into awareness.

The third thing in rebirthing is to stay awake. At night, you breathe deeply and relax, and you sleep. Sleeping is not rebirthing and it's not transformative.

The fourth thing is an attitude of acceptance, recognising that everything that is happening during the rebirthing session reflects your conscious and unconscious mind. By accepting this, you lessen the chance that your conditioning might mask an important insight.

Sandra lay down on the bed. I covered her with a blanket and she started to breathe as I turned on an *Enya* CD. During the first ten minutes, she relaxed, and her breathing became deeper and more rhythmical. After about twenty minutes of connected breathing, her cheeks flushed, the breathing was labouring, hands were tightening up and she was becoming tense. This tension continued for about a further fifteen minutes before she released it. The breathing returned to normal, the hands softened, and she looked peaceful. I said she could stop the connected breathing and rest for a few minutes.

In her debrief afterwards, Sandra said had felt very tight and tingly in the hands, had become very hot and remembered an incident as a child with her grandmother who had been living with her family. Her pet rabbit had died; Gran had told her not to be stupid and to stop crying. She had told Sandra's mother that she was spoiling the child by comforting her. In Sandra's family, as a child, she was discouraged from showing any feelings.

Consequently, as an adult Sandra found it difficult to express her feelings and did not know how to communicate what she really thought. She often put up with situations she did not like. This had resulted in her becoming emotionally constipated. She had no way of releasing her tension, and this in turn had developed into panic attacks. Stored anxiety is like a bomb. All the emotions that are felt and not expressed are stored in the body waiting for something to trigger them until the person 'explodes'.

After the initial rebirthing, Sandra experienced an immediate easing of the stress she had been carrying. Over the next ten months, she saw me for another twelve sessions, gradually feeling calmer and more confident. The frequency and severity of the anxiety diminished. As well as releasing the pent-up emotions, Sandra also changed her behaviour and attitude towards expressing her feelings. Two years after the initial series of consultations, Sandra had not had a re-occurrence of the panic attacks.

Rebirthing uses the breath to vitalise and energise the body, emotions and mind. As the body is energised, past memories and emotions are reactivated, reconceptualised and released. If this process is taken far enough, there is a new orientation for the personality, a new sense of identity. The long-term goal for rebirthing, after the transforming of the pain and conditioning, is to experience a profound state of meditation.

Rebirthing was rediscovered by Leonard Orr in the early 1970's, while meditating in a hot tub he had a spontaneous healing release. Initially he thought it was the hot water in the tub that was the key factor, later he realised it was the breathing. Nowadays, most rebirthing takes place on a bed with the rebirther, (the client) being supported by a rebirthing practitioner.

Leonard called the breathing technique rebirthing because he believed to heal the personality you had to release and re-experience your birth memory, and with the letting go of the old emotional and mental conditioning, you are symbolically reborn.

> ...as the body is energised, past memories and emotions are reactivated, reconceptualised and released...

The personality of your parents and the experiences during the first seven years of life are also significant factors that determine personality. In addition to this, many people have an easy and loving birth and don't have any traumatic birth memory to release. Other names for rebirthing are Holotropic Breathing, Vivation, Breathworks, Conscious Connected Breathing and Breath Therapy.

The technique has a very long history as it was used by the ancient yogis of India. On several trips to India, Leonard Orr, under the instructions of his teacher Babaji, refined and simplified the technique. The mystic alchemists of the Middle-

Ages also used a similar breathing technique to 'strip the base metal (the ego) of its dross and transform it to gold (spirit)'.

Rebirthing's primary benefit is to release and re-balance the emotions. Almost any condition where you feel stressed, overemotional or incomplete can be released with rebirthing.

Michael Adamedes has been a psychotherapist and rebirther practitioner for more than 35 years. For more information regarding private consultations and Rebirth Breathing Retreats, go to: michaeladamedes.com

REFLEXOLOGY

Reflexology is a crafted combination of finger and thumb techniques applied primarily to the feet, hands and/or ears to activate and awaken the body's own healing powers to restore and balance our organs, glands and body area functions.

The feet, hands and ears all represent a map of our body: toes/fingers represent head and neck areas; ball of foot/upper palm the chest area; arch of foot/ lower palm the abdomen, digestive areas; heel /base of hand relates to the pelvis area. The spine is located on the inside areas of the foot and the outside thumb to wrist area of the hands.

Each reflexologist develops their own unique symposium from many studied philosophies to collate the best suited treatment for your requirements. With 75% of dis-ease being related to stress of some degree, reflexology can help provide a relaxation effect to assist the equilibrium of the body's function. When the body rests, it can begin to restore itself physically,

> *When the body rests it can begin to restore itself physically, psychologically and spiritually.*

psychologically and spiritually. Coping in today's world can bring many personal challenges leading to depression, anxiety, helplessness and substance abuse, to name a few which impacts on our daily function level.

Working within this field for a number of years, it is always humbling when these clients having received reflexology, say "I feel good now" and their facial expressions are relaxed and happy. Relief for 20-30 mins or up to one day provides hope for their life, when they are challenged daily just to function.

One client who was extensively agitated in a group session was taken aside to work with the counsellor. I arrived during this time and waited to give the scheduled treatment. They were very grateful I had waited and said they felt okay, but I could tell by the clenched fists that maybe things weren't quite worked through! The client got up on table and no conversation took place as I gently worked to relax and nurture through the reflexology techniques. I left the room to wash my hands while the client got up and put their shoes and socks back on. On returning, I noticed the clients' facial expression was bewilderment/amazement and they said, "Now I know reflexology works. I was not in a good space when you started, and I am so relaxed now and all my anger and agitation has gone.'

Now, that's what inspires me to continue!

Karen Waimana, **Aroam'n Reflexology**
Medical Intuitive (Professional Member of International Institute of Medical Intuitives), Reflexologist (Life Member Reflexology New Zealand Inc), Aromatherapist (Diploma in Aromatherapy), Natural Perfume Training(Level 2 USA), Healing Touch Practitioner Training

Ph: 64274197640 Email: aroamnkaren@gmail.com
Facebook: Karen Waimana
www.aroamnreflexology.nz

SLEEP

Sleep is fundamental to life. Sleep is essential for the proper functioning of the body and the mind. Without adequate, restful sleep, the body will experience sleep deprivation. This will result in a decreased ability to concentrate, perform complex tasks, communicate and listen effectively.

> *Sleep is essential for the proper functioning of the body and the mind.*

Sufficient sleep is 5-10 hours a night depending on the individual needs. Most people will sleep an average of 8 hours. Children usually need 10-12 hours for growth, whereas the elderly usually survive happily on 5-6 hours a night.

Anyone who is unwell or recovering from illness requires more sleep rest as this allows for the body to grow, repair, recuperate and revitalise. A major contributor to sleep is the circadian rhythm. This is a 24-hour cycle. This is divided into REM (rapid eye movement) and NREM (non-rapid eye movement). NREM sleep is known as 'quiet sleep'. It is a time of slow measured breathing, some snoring and very little body movement. In this state, our senses are least responsive.

In REM sleep, snoring stops, breathing becomes erratic, and facial and fingertip muscles may twitch; dreaming may occur. A standard night's sleep of eight hours is usually divided into four or five cycles of ninety minutes. In a cycle of ninety minutes, you experience four stages of sleep before you go onto the next ninety-minute cycle, or you wake. The body and brain are designed to sleep at night and work in the day. This is how you function at your best and are most productive.

There are many people who work in much needed service industries which include nursing, medical, police, emergency, transport, mining, firefighters, ambulance, bakery and flight staff that do night duty and suffer with sleep disorders.

In 1997 in Helsinki, a heart study was conducted over five years on the Finnish population, which revealed that people who worked night duty showed a 50% increase in heart disease compared to day shift workers. Other ailments prone to night duty are: fatigue, high blood pressure, diarrhoea, constipation, abdominal pain, weight gain, peptic ulcers, gastrointestinal upsets and sleep disorders.

According to Josling, *Shift Work and Ill-health*, 1999, other social and physiological issues from sleep deprivation include depression (due to a drop-in dopamine and serotonin - the hormones that make you feel good), irritability, poor judgment, high divorce rates, an increased incidence of accidents and a higher degree of substance abuse. Most people on night duty view their work as stressful.

Working night duty for twelve years myself, I found that night duty became a lifestyle and I needed to operate in a certain way to get the best out of nights and the best out of myself. I noted that many staff working nights tend to do the following to 'just to stay awake and keep moving': frequent cigarette breaks, drinking copious amounts of coffee or Coca-Cola and eating foods high in carbohydrates and sugar. All these practices give you the 'buzz' effect which gets you through the night, but unfortunately have a detrimental effect on the body and your sleep process.

> *Cigarettes, coffee and Coca-Cola dehydrate you, which compromises the immune system...*

Cigarettes, coffee and Coca-Cola dehydrate you, which compromises the immune system, and carbohydrates and sugar promote mood fluctuations. It takes the body 48 hours to fully readjust and recover after a stretch of night duty.

Tips for night duty
Ideally, if you can sleep well in the day, then night shift may be suited to you. If not, then limit the amount of nights you do.

- Eat your main meal 2-3 hours before start of shift, this will give you energy for the night.
- If you eat on night duty the hours of 10pm and 2am are best.
- Eat 2-3 hours before sleep or on waking.
- Your digestion may change on night duty so light meals and warm soups may be indicated.
- A normal sleep on nights is usually 4-6 hours. The body will catch up on any sleep deficiency when you have days off.
- Regular exercise, dance and/or yoga help the body to sleep.
- If you suffer with constipation due to irregular digestion, make sure your diet is high in fibre, fruits and water.
- Avoid dry chips and dry foods as they aggravate constipation.
- If working in air-conditioning, you may suffer with dehydration.
- Maintaining high fluid intake and applying cream to hands and face will keep the body moist.
- Have 15-20 minutes of sun daily or take a Vitamin D supplement.
- Tell people you are sleeping in the day and turn all your phones, faxes and answering machine off, on silent mode or reduced volume.

- Sleep in a cool, dark room. Use a fan if it is hot in summer.
- Use earplugs to minimise noise and nightshades to reduce light.
- Avoid chocolate, coffee, Coca-Cola and junk food as they act as stimulants making it more difficult to sleep.
- If you drink juice at night, dilute it with water (50/50) as juice is mainly sugar which interferes with sleep.
- If you are prone to eating breakfast before you sleep you may gain weight as digestion is slow when you sleep.
- Eating fruit one hour before sleep is fine as fruit is easily digested.
- If you are in a seated profession and suffer with lower back pain, rolling a warm towel and placing it at your lower back will maintain its own body alignment. Always use a straight-backed chair to support your back.
- Avoid ice and all cold foods and fluids as this slows down digestion which could lead to constipation.
- If feeling tired while driving home, take ice cubes and suck on them. This will wake up your senses.
- Take time to unwind when you get home.
- Sleep to soft music.
- You often get a second wind when you leave work, so use this time and energy to pay bills and do shopping.

Tips during night-shift duty

- Eat light meals for easy digestion while on nights.
- 5-6 hours' sleep in the day is sufficient, this is normal.
- Maintain regular exercise.
- Do yoga to empty stomach and bowels.
- Keep bowels regular; add fibre to diet if indicated.
- Maintain hydration 2-3 litres; no coffee, cola or fizzy drinks.
- Warm soups, Khichadi and juice go well on night duty.

- If eating on night duty, the best time is from 10pm to 2am.
- Daily exposure to sunlight, about 15 minutes helps normalise the body.
- Turn off all phones and tell people you are sleeping in the day, so you are not disturbed.
- Sleep in a dark, warm room with earplugs and nightshades.
- No breakfast before bed (fruit is ok) as you will gain weight.
- No ice, cold drinks, dairy, carbohydrates, chocolate or raw foods.

Suggested foods to increase dopamine and serotonin

Dopamine and serotonin are our 'happy' hormones. When working nightshift, these hormone levels drop due to irregular sleep patterns. As a result, you may experience mood fluctuations and depression.

The following are foods which help maintain dopamine and serotonin levels and it is recommended to eat these foods when you get hungry through the night:

Apples, avocado, bananas, almonds, brazil nuts, cashews, hazelnuts, walnuts, pistachios, beans, lima beans, beets, celery, pineapple, watermelon, green leafy vegetables, potato, radish, tomato, cheese, cottage cheese, chicken, turkey, cucumber, figs, fish, mackerel, sardines, tuna, ham, honey, milk, eggs, tofu, wholegrain, yoghurt, brown rice, pasta, sesame seeds and pumpkin seeds.

TAI CHI

Tai Chi in its most traditional form, is the classic martial art. Although many of the movements are the same, the underlying intent of attack and defence has been modified when you undertake Tai Chi for health and well-being. Most teachers and masters teach Tai Chi Chuan. Chuan in this sense, is the *form,* whereas Tai Chi is the inner place which transcends form and the effort to achieve it. It is not about finding a good teacher – it is an aha! – finding it within yourself.

Practised in this way, Tai Chi has a lot to offer. One of the major benefits is to restore confidence in the way you move your body and the control you have over it. Watch children play. They run backwards without looking. They balance with poise on one leg with arms out-flung. We forget that those skills are ours, no matter what our age. All we can do is to claim them back.

> ...*Tai Chi puts you in balance, and when we are in balance we function in a harmonious way.*

Because it is based on the natural flows and rhythms of the body, Tai Chi puts you in balance, and when we are in balance we function in a harmonious way. This harmony is evident in both our innermost private self as well as our outer public persona.

Tai Chi awakens you - keeps you centred and connected with your surroundings. It is not a *series of poses,* it is a movement *pattern* – pattern, not form.

We are used to thinking of our centre as being fixed, as in yoga or meditation, but Tai Chi is mastery of the moving centre. The outside/inside awareness – not the inner focus of meditation. A place where you don't think – the movement just happens.

To get to that place, of course, takes a bit of time and like any other skill, you need to learn the basics. Learning anything new can cause us to concentrate intently and tense up. The aim however, is to get past that awkward phase as soon as possible, to become resilient and responsive.

As you work, you use the form, or the pattern as a guide. It is something to work with – a process which serves you. No matter what Tai Chi looks like from the outside - a pattern or a structure - what is happening inside the body is very different. Tai Chi is neither set structure, nor chaos. It is a different kind of organisation which cannot be known just by learning a set of patterned movements. If this was what Tai Chi was all about, you would get bored and stuck in repetition, the result of not being taught properly. It is one thing to learn *the form* – it is another to get the origin first – the spontaneous, creative process. We aim to be able to relate to the basic underlying art rather than become a robot by concentrating on meticulous details. It's all about subtlety.

> Tai Chi is neither set structure, nor chaos.

When you get it, it looks like you made it up on the spot. There is a continuity of letting one movement lead smoothly into another without any breaks, hesitations or sudden changes.

Steve Martin sees the innate balance in Tai Chi thus:

"If I continually reach out to others for love, I am tipping forward, off centre and unstable, leaning on whoever I contact and likely to fall flat and hard if the other leaves. If I continually withdraw in fear I am tipping backward, tense and rigid and the slightest surprise will push me over. If I feel uncertain and unstable in my base, then all my

contacts with others will be wobbly and lack conviction. In contrast, if I can become centred and balanced in my own experience, then I can carry this moving centre with me. If I am balanced now, then I can move in any direction I wish, with no danger of falling. My contact with others is solid and real, coming to you from the root of my being."

There are many reported health benefits from doing Tai Chi as your regular form of exercise. These include improvements to your energy levels, sleeping better, more flexibility and endurance, improved circulation of the blood, increase immunity, reduction of pain, less craving for salty and sweet foods. These are physical responses, but there are also psychological benefits with improvement to mood, confidence and self-esteem, less stress being some the positive changes people have reported. It is specifically advised for arthritis, diabetes and people in need of gentle strengthening. As a bonus, there is the possibility of a reduced need for other therapies. New research reveals that there is some evidence that Tai Chi may help the brain-function of people who are experiencing impairment to their cognitive ability after chemotherapy.

The recommendation is to attend two classes a week, with three sessions of practice at home for those who are wanting to do Tai Chi as part of a health program. Like any other exercise, it is wise to incorporate it into your life plan and to do it regularly and consistently. Tai Chi involves so many parts of the body and helps to relax the mind, which makes it more likely that participants will stay with their program.

To move with grace, power and beauty, to harmonise with the heartbeat, the breath and the universe is to receive the greatest gift that Tai Chi offers.

Presented by Suzanne May, Tai Chi Instructor

TISSUE SALTS

Tissue Salts, also known as Cell Salts, have been a part of medical science in Europe since the early 1800's. However, their significance has been known in India since Vedic times, dating back five thousand years.

Dr Wilhelm Heinrich Schuessler, a notable doctor, homeopath, physiological chemist, and physicist, dedicated himself to identifying a simple unified system to explain them. Because of his research and experiments, he established the twelve cell salts necessary for normal cell function and the maintenance of good health.

Tissue Salts are inorganic minerals that are part of our cells. Every cell contains many of these salts, which are needed to maintain balance within our body. The health of our cells is directly linked to wellbeing and disease. If these cell salts are deficient, signs and symptoms will occur and if not correctly treated, will eventually lead to disease.

> *Tissue salts are inorganic minerals... which are needed to maintain balance within our body.*

Tissue Salts perform a vital role in body maintenance, such as:

- Body metabolism e.g. acid-alkaline homoeostasis.
- Providing strength and rigidity to bones.
  Giving support to building muscle, cartilage and blood cells.
- Aiding in digestion and elimination.
- Assisting in production of saliva and digestive juices.

- Excellent for growing children (there is entire range especially for children).

To determine which tissue salts are lacking, it is necessary to identify symptoms and the part of the body affected. Specific tissues salts and minerals are more likely to be deficient at various stages of a person's life. These can be determined by a Medical Astrologer.

Tissue salts can be used in conjunction with prescribed medications and should be taken between meals without any fluid, or as prescribed on the bottle. They should be dissolved under the tongue and are sweet tasting.

Tissue salts are usually made in a milk-lactose base (important to check the bottle), so individuals allergic to milk or lactose DO NOT take unless under medical supervision. Tissue salts also come in a spray formulation.

Fiona's Story

In 2010, I slipped on a puddle of water and tore the lateral ligaments of my left knee. After a night at work, I couldn't weight-bear as my knee had swollen. The physiotherapist recommended resting my knee for one week on crutches, along with the usual ultrasound treatment. As a working mother and solo parent with four children, it wasn't financially viable for me to be off work for a long period of time.

On the advice of a Medical Astrologer, I commenced taking tissue salts Calc Phos and Mag Phos alternately every hour while awake. The second week I took Calc Flour and Kali Mur every hour. The Physio was surprised at the speed of recovery and the mobility and strength I regained in such a brief time. I returned to yoga within three weeks, was back at work within a week and avoided surgery. A win-win situation.

WATSU®

Imagine an indulgent spa-like experience where you are floated in warm water. Floating on your back, you let the water support you, taking away your aches and pains. The combination of the warm water (~35C) and the rhythmic movement slows the breath and stressors melt away. Dynamic movement patterns and the friction and viscosity of the water provide rocking and stretches, stimulating and opening the body. Interspersed are moments of stillness supported in nurturing holds.

At times, you feel you are in your mother's womb or perhaps a ballerina, or seaweed on a reef feeling the undulation and rush of the waves. Or, as one client felt, "I'm a mermaid spaceman."

Maybe you are here for the unique water experience or perhaps you are seeking the benefits of pain relief, deep relaxation, or to release physical or emotional blockages. Either way, you are experiencing Watsu® or one of the related aquatic bodywork techniques such as WaterDance®, Healing Dance®, or Aquatic Integration®. Watsu® comes from the words water + shiatsu. Besides point work and holds there is joint mobilisation and stretching all while being moved through three dimensions (or even four if you consider both above and below the surface of the water).

Watsu® is performed in one-on-one pool sessions in chest-deep warm water. For most sessions, the receiver (client) floats on their back with their face

Research is finding value of Watsu® with individuals of Post-Traumatic Stress Disorder...

out of the water. The practitioner lightly supports the receiver's head and lower torso allowing the buoyancy of water to provide most of the support. Floats may be attached to the legs to increase floatation in some individuals. This is important for good body alignment. As the comfort level and trust increases, the receiver let's go and does nothing. The practitioner looks as if they are going through a Tai Qi form with someone in their arms. Fluid movements while holding one leg or arm, bringing knees to chest while pivoting through the water, and other endless manipulations provide openings, closings, spirals, and more.

If receiver is keen, an underwater session can be explored. Using nose plugs and signals between provider and receiver, a whole new dimension of bodywork is on offer. Whether you have the sense of a jellyfish, a sea anemone, a dolphin, or a complete fetal inversion, it is a complete new world. Many clients find it especially freeing and a space and time to release grief and address personal issues. Research is finding value of Watsu® with individuals with post-traumatic stress disorder (PTSD) and Jennifer has noted increased value with the underwater work with these clients.

Individuals report a range of benefits. Relief from various symptoms often occur, these effects are coincidental with the relaxation, release, and balancing effects of Watsu® and related techniques. Perhaps you would like to experience? We'd love for you to join us in the water.

The Worldwide Aquatic Association oversees training programs for Watsu® and related aquatic bodywork modalities. WABA also maintains an official registry of certified practitioners and instructors, classes, and training institutes around the world. The Aquatic Bodywork Association of New Zealand has a WABA approved training path and list of practitioners at www.watsu.org.nz ABANZ is an affiliate of Natural Health Practitioners of New Zealand.

Jennifer Leaf, MSc is a Registered Watsu® Practitioner (WABA and Aquatic Bodywork Association New Zealand) with training in Healing Dance® and Aquatic Integration®. She practices in Napier, Hawke's Bay from her private heated pool. Her website is www.qiworks.nz or email her at jleaf@qiworks.nz or 021 298 6740.

YOGA

Yoga is a state of being. It is about oneness with ourselves and everything else in the cosmos of which we are a part. Obtaining this state of enlightenment and self-realisation can happen over many lifetimes or in an instant, but this still doesn't tell us what it is. It is an experienced state to be felt, smelt, expressed, and embodied. But what is it like? It is like being you without all the accumulated habits, held experiences and layers of identity - basically it is existence as our essence, the nature of

> ...as our body becomes lighter and less bound by accumulated blockages, we begin to reclaim our birth-right, our happiness...

which is joy. This is not the '*you*' who goes to the shops, goes to work, or is partner, parent, singer, charity worker etc. When you take away all those layers of accumulated thoughts and patterns that are woven into a cloak of identity, there is the essence of '*you*' that was born to this planet and the '*you*' that will go beyond it.

When we practice yoga in class, at home or out in the world, we practice being our true selves. This practice can incorporate any practice of the eight limbs of yoga as outlined in Patanjali's Yoga Sutras. For example, in asana practice (physical postures) we bend our body into specific shapes, angles and triangles that open channels in our bodies and adjust our nervous, glandular, digestive, urinary, cardiovascular, musculoskeletal and sensory systems. We also align muscles, joints, ligaments and encourage healthy organ function and tissue and cell regeneration. Even though we focus on or isolate parts of our bodies in a posture, the whole of us is receiving some effect; this includes our mind, energy system, emotions and spirit.

When we combine specific physical yoga practices for a cleansing effect, we create a kriya. Kundalini Yoga as taught by Yogi Bhajan is one yoga lineage that uses the technology of kriya. Kundalini Yoga is much more than just a system of physical exercises. It is a dynamic, powerful tool for expanding awareness. It is particularly useful for cleansing and freeing ourselves on many levels from toxins and blockages we have accumulated in day-to-day life experience through our patterns or habits but may also have carried into this lifetime as samskaras (karmic imprints).

As our body becomes lighter and less bound by accumulated blockages, we begin to reclaim our birthright, our happiness. This is often when we catch a glimpse of what yoga is all about - living in our true state of happiness and connection with all that exists. The Master of Kundalini Yoga explains: "You should make yourself so happy that by looking at you, other people become happy" - Yogi Bhajan.

Aleta Lafferty has been fascinated by the mystical from an early age and began studying and teaching various forms of meditation and kundalini yoga in her 20s to Sydney's Newtown community. She is now a working mum of two and meditating away to keep the balance between the city and the stars. You can read more or contact her at aletalafferty.tumblr.com

Personal Notes

Glossary

Ama - a toxic by-product generated by incomplete digestion

Apana – downward movement of prana

Astrology – study of the cosmos; how it affects human lives

Ayurveda – the science of life

Babaji – Guru or teacher

Central Nervous System – controls functions in body & mind

Chakra – wheel of life; subtle body energy centre. There are seven chakras:
1. Muladhara – located base of spine
2. Svadhisthana – located between in the sacral area
3. Manipura – located above the naval
4. Anahata – located in the chest
5. Vishuddha – located in the throat
6. Ajna – located between the eyebrows
7. Sahasrara – located on top of the head

DHEAS – Dehydroepiandrosterone – a hormone

Dinacharya – daily routine

Dopamine – neurotransmitter in the brain that motivates

Dosha – a biological element. There are 3 Doshas:
1. Vata – governs all movement in the bodymind
2. Pitta – governs metabolism in the bodymind
3. Kapha – governs structure in the bodymind

Endocrine System – glands that produce hormones

Energy Field – connects the etheric to the physical body. The higher the level the closer to self-actualisation:
1. Etheric or vital – closest to the physical body
2. Emotional – carries unresolved emotions
3. Mental – carries all thought forms
4. Intuitive or astral – links intuition & cognition
5. Etheric template – connects to sound
6. Celestial body – soul essence
7. Ketheric body – connects universal consciousness

Horoscope – hour of watching

Karma – law of cause and effect

Kundalini – primal energy located at the base of the spine

Marma Chikitsa – points on the body influencing energy flow

Metaphysics – philosophy dealing with abstract concepts

Muscle Testing – diagnosis based on muscle strength

Ojas – a healthy Dosha

Prana – the lifeforce (the breath)

Pranayama – the control of breath

Rasayana - rejuvenation

Ritucharya – seasonal routine

Samana – horizontal movement of prana

Serotonin – neurological hormone affecting mood

Soul Direction – spiritual pathway

Spiritual Wellness – purposeful life to balance soul & body

Tejas – type of energy or vitality

Udana – upward movement of prana

Vyana – prana around the body

In gratitude and with many thanks...

I would like to acknowledge and express my appreciation to all those people who helped me make this book possible.

To those who contributed their expertise through the voice of their articles, I applaud you all in your life's work and thank you for your knowledge.

Individually they are:
Michael Adamedes for his amazing work in Rebirthing;
thanks to Shirley Arbuckle Hart and Roslyn Hart, The Ayurvedic Institute, Albuquerque, NM: www.ayurveda.com;
Amalia Cardile, Massage Therapist with the golden hands;
Farida Irania for her wisdom and Bowen therapy;
Maggie Kerr, my Astrological Psychological Mentor;
Professor Dr P H Kulkarni, Father of Ayurveda;
Aleta Lafferty, Yoga Instructor extraordinaire;
Angela Hair, Homeopathy;
Jennifer Leaf, soothing Watsu® Therapist Instructor;
Jennabeth Moss, my soul sister in meditation;
Dr Rama Prasad, Ayurvedic Mentor;
Susanne May, graceful Tai Chi Instructor;
Charlotte Mildon, Māori Healer;
Dr Chris Tsioutis, exceptional Alternative Medical Practitioner;
Karen Waimana, Reflexologist;
Rachel Wright, Intuitive Naturopath; and, from Sydney,
www.facebook.com/YogainDailyLifeSydney
www.yogaindailylife.org.au/Sydney

To Fiona Campbell, Louise Kesterson and to those who wished to remain anonymous, I thank you for your support by contributing your personal stories.

Last, but by no means least, to Win Needham my manuscript assessor from Inklings: Professional Proofreading & Editing Services. Without her writing skills and creative computer expertise, I could not have completed my vision. To you my friend, my deepest and warmest appreciation.

Photograph of Christina on back cover © 2016 Bauermedia.

White light
PUBLISHING HOUSE

www.ingramcontent.com/pod-product-compliance
Lightning Source LLC
Chambersburg PA
CBHW071911290426
44110CB00013B/1350